Current Practice in Health Sciences Librarianship

Alison Bunting

Editor-in-Chief

Volume 3
Information Access and Delivery in Health Sciences Libraries

Edited by
Carolyn E. Lipscomb

Medical Library Association
and
The Scarecrow Press, Inc.
Lanham, Md. & London

British Library Cataloguing-in-Publication data available

Library of Congress Cataloging-in-Publication Data

Information access and delivery in health sciences libraries / edited
by Carolyn E. Lipscomb.
      p. cm. — (Current practice in health sciences librarianship ;
v. 3)
    Includes index.
    ISBN 0-8108-3050-7 (alk. paper)
    1. Medical libraries—United States. 2. Libraries—United States—
Circulation, loans. 3. Bibliographical services—United States.
4. Interlibrary loans—United States. I. Lipscomb, Carolyn E.
II. Series.
    [DNLM: 1. Library services—organization & administration—
United States. Z 675.M4 C976 1996 v.3]
Z675.M4I43 1996
026.61'0973—dc20
DNLM/DLC
for Library of Congress   95-42302

Information Access and Delivery in
Health Sciences Libraries

Contents

Preface

Current Practice in Health Sciences Librarianship (CPHSL) continues the publication principles established by its predecessor, the *Handbook of Medical Library Practice*, to serve as: a general introduction to the field of health sciences librarianship for graduate students; a source of basic information and references to the literature for the Medical Library Association's (MLA) professional development and recognition program; a reference work for health sciences librarians and other information specialists, providing basic information in areas peripheral to their own expertise; and a means of documenting the state of practice of health sciences librarianship at a particular point in time.

The decision to change the title of this venerable MLA publication is best explained by a review of the *Handbook*'s publication history. The appearance in 1942 of the first edition of the *Handbook,* published by the American Library Association, fulfilled a long-standing goal of the MLA. As editor Janet Doe noted,

> The demand [for a Handbook] has grown keener with the passage of time, undoubtedly because of the recent rapid increase in the number of medical libraries, for half of the 315 now existing in this country have originated since 1910. To staff these libraries, workers have been enticed or commandeered from general and special libraries, from library schools, from the clerical staff of hospitals or medical schools, and from doctors' offices [1].

The second edition of the *Handbook* (1956), edited by Janet Doe and Mary Louise Marshall [2], updated the one-volume first edition, retaining, whenever possible, the original chapter authors. The preface to this volume included an apology for publication delays and noted that some of the information in the volume was written three or more years prior to publication.

Fourteen years elapsed before the third edition, the first one published by MLA, appeared in 1970. Editors Gertrude L. Annan and Jacqueline W. Felter took an entirely different approach: "The chapters are written by a new cadre of authors and differ from those of the earlier edition in substance and emphasis"[3]. Despite the expansion of the scope and coverage, the one-volume format was retained. Four consultants from different types of health sciences libraries ensured that the content took into account library practice in these settings. Publication delays continued to be a problem and were

> ...of grave concern to the editors who regret that some chapters were written several years before the volume went to press. With so many involved in the preparation of the work, unforeseen emergencies arose which prevented its production in the period scheduled [4].

Louise Darling, David Bishop, and Lois Ann Colaianni edited the fourth edition, published between 1982 and 1988. This edition included a "...shift in terminology from medical to health science libraries...in itself...indicative of the new complexity, the highly interdisciplinary nature of the fields served by these libraries"[5]. However, the title of the *Handbook* was not changed "...because of the risk of obscuring the continuity of editions"[6]. A three-volume format was chosen to: "...accommodate material on new developments, lessen the delays inherent in a multiple-author work, and facilitate later revision..."[7]. This new approach did not, however, prevent publication delays

> ...even with a smaller number of authors per volume, the considerable time difference in submission of chapters has meant that the problem of keeping material within the volume on the same level of currency, though reduced, has not been solved [8].

And, "...the sequential publication has resulted in problems of uneven currency in the completed work . . ."[9]. "A more satisfactory method for revising the *Handbook* in the future is now under study, as the rapid pace of change in the information field obviously requires a new approach"[10].

In 1989, the MLA Books Panel recommended that the *Handbook* be continued with the same general scope and content as the fourth edition, but that the three volumes be further divided into a series of smaller monographs, each dealing with a single subject and each with its own volume editor. An editor-in-chief, assisted by an Advisory Committee, was appointed to coordinate the publication.

The Advisory Committee determined that health sciences librarianship is changing so rapidly that the profession will be better served by publication of a series, and that the series required a new title. In this way, individual volumes can be updated as needed, without having to wait for the completion of all volumes in an edition, and the individual volumes will have a greater identity as independent books.

CPHSL will appear in eight volumes. The editors are noted below:

Volume 1: Reference and Information Services in Health Sciences Libraries, *M. Sandra Wood, editor*

Volume 2: Educational Services in Health Sciences Libraries, *Francesca Allegri, editor*

Volume 3: Information Access and Delivery in Health Sciences Libraries, *Carolyn E. Lipscomb, editor*

Volume 4: Collection Development and Assessment in Health Sciences Libraries, *Dottie Eakin and Daniel T. Richards*

Volume 5: Acquisitions in Health Sciences Libraries, *David Morse, editor*

Volume 6: Bibliographic Management of Information Resources in Health Sciences Libraries, *Laurie L. Thompson, editor*

Volume 7: Health Sciences Environment and Librarianship in Health Sciences Libraries, *Lucretia W. McClure, editor*

Volume 8: Administration and Management in Health Sciences Libraries, *Rick B. Forsman, editor*

The editor-in-chief is extremely fortunate in being able to tap the expertise of a group of very talented and dedicated MLA members as advisors, editors, and chapter authors. The *CPHSL* Advisory Committee provided valuable advice on the organization and content of *CPHSL*, recommended a publication plan and timetable, and assisted in the identification of editors and chapter authors.

The editors have total responsibility for the preparation for publication of their volume, including selection of authors, review of content and adherence to established style and format guidelines, and maintenance of the publication schedule. Authors were asked to include in their chapters, as applicable, the following considerations: ethics, standards, legal aspects, staffing issues and implications, differing practices as they apply to different types of libraries, research, evaluation, technology/automation, and budgeting and financing.

An extensive expert review process involved both academic and hospital librarians. Each volume includes a listing of the expert reviewers in grateful acknowledgment of their efforts. The editor-in-chief and the editors are indebted to MLA's Managing Editor of Books, J. Michael Homan, for selecting reviewers and coordinating their work, and for his personal suggestions on organization, content, and format.

CPHSL is co-published by the Medical Library Association and Scarecrow Press, Inc. Special thanks are due to David B. Biesel, Director of Scarecrow's Association Publishing Program, Raymond S. Naegele, MLA's Director of Financial and Administrative Services, and Kimberly S. Pierceall, MLA's Director of Communications, for their advice and assistance. The indexing expertise of Beryl Glitz provides consistent and accurate access to the content of each volume.

Alison Bunting, Editor-in-Chief
Louise M. Darling Biomedical Library
University of California, Los Angeles

References

1. Doe J, ed. Handbook of medical library practice. Chicago: American Library Association, 1942:v.

2. Doe J, Marshall ML, eds. Handbook of medical library practice. 2nd ed. Chicago: American Library Association, 1956.

3. Annan GL, Felter JW, eds. Handbook of medical library practice. 3rd ed. Chicago: Medical Library Association, 1970:v.

4. Ibid., vii.

5. Darling L, Bishop D, Colaianni LA, eds. Handbook of medical library practice. 4th ed. vol. 1. Chicago: Medical Library Association, 1982: xi.

6. Ibid.

7. Ibid., xii.

8. Darling L, Bishop D, Colaianni LA, eds. Handbook of medical library practice. 4th ed. vol. 3. Chicago: Medical Library Association, 1988:xiv.

9. Ibid.

10. Ibid., xv.

Expert Reviewers

Margaret Bandy, Denver, CO
Rya Ben-Shir, Berwyn, IL
Eloise C. Foster, Chicago, IL
Nelson J. Gilman, Los Angeles, CA
Cynthia H. Goldstein, New Orleans, LA
Gretchen Hallerberg, Cleveland, OH
Brett A. Kirkpatrick, Galveston, TX
Lucretia W. McClure, Rochester, NY
T. Scott Plutchak, St. Louis, MO
Peter Stangl, Stanford, CA
Mary Edith Walker, Memphis, TN
Carolyn G. Weaver, Seattle, WA

Advisory Committee Members

Rachael K. Anderson
Director, Health Sciences Center Library
University of Arizona
Tucson, AZ

Alison Bunting
Associate University Librarian for Sciences
Louise Darling Biomedical Library
University of California, Los Angeles
Los Angeles, CA

Dottie Eakin
Director, Medical Sciences Library
Texas A&M University
College Station, TX

Rick Forsman
Director, Denison Memorial Library
University of Colorado Health Sciences Center
Denver, CO

Ruth Holst
Director of Library Services
Medical Library
Columbia Hospital
Milwaukee, WI

J. Michael Homan
Director of Libraries
Mayo Foundation
Rochester, MN

Mary Horres
Associate University Librarian for Sciences
Biomedical Library
University of California, San Diego
La Jolla, CA

Kimberly Pierceall
Director of Communications
Medical Library Association
Chicago, IL

M. Sandra Wood
Librarian, Reference and Database Services
George T. Harrell Library
Milton S. Hershey Medical Center
Pennsylvania State University
Hershey, PA

Authors

Gretchen Naisawald Arnold
Associate Director for Public Services
Claude Moore Health Sciences Library
University of Virginia Medical Center
Charlottesville, VA

James Curtis
Assistant Director for Information and Education Services
Health Sciences Library
University of North Carolina
Chapel Hill, NC

Martha R. Fishel
Deputy Chief
Public Services Division
National Library of Medicine
Bethesda, MD

Beryl Glitz
Associate Director
Pacific Southwest Regional Medical Library
UCLA Louise Darling Biomedical Library
Los Angeles, CA

Susan Russell Lessick
Head of Research and Instructional Services
Science Library
University of California, Irvine
Irvine, CA

Carolyn E. Lipscomb
Consultant
Durham, NC

Irene Lovas
Network Coordinator
Pacific Southwest Regional Medical Library
UCLA Louise Darling Biomedical Library
Los Angeles, CA

Valerie L. Su
Deputy Director and Head of Public Services
Lane Medical Library
Stanford University Medical Center
Stanford, CA

N.J. Wolfe
Associate Director for Information Services
Ehrman Medical Library
New York University Medical Center
New York, NY

Introduction

Trends in Access and Delivery

This volume addresses information access and delivery in health sciences libraries through examination of circulation, interlibrary loan and document delivery, and fee-based services. The discussion of these topics illustrates both the unique aspects of health sciences libraries as well as their commonality with all types of libraries. Access and delivery in health sciences libraries are being shaped by the same strong environmental forces which are reverberating in libraries and information in general. Historically, health sciences libraries have played a pioneering role in using technology to improve access to information; today they continue to lead in areas such as automated document delivery systems.

As Alison Bunting pointed out in her Janet Doe Lecture to the Medical Library Association, changes in the health sciences librarian profession can be identified through examination of the first four editions of the *Handbook of Medical Library Practice* and its successor *Current Practice in Health Sciences Librarianship* [1]. She traced trends in access and delivery through the decades including the growth in service and increased focus on these functions, the addition of new formats, and the impact of automation. Automation of identification, request and transmission mechanisms, and enhanced cooperation promoted by the Regional Medical Library Program were remarkable changes which improved the ability of health sciences libraries to provide accurate and speedy delivery of material. Legal, policy, and economic considerations also became increasingly important [2].

Information access and delivery services in health sciences libraries today are in transition. The trends noted by Bunting continue to affect methods of providing traditional access and delivery. Advances in technology and the development of systems offer many opportunities for improving the management of access to local resources and of delivery of information among libraries and from other external sources. These same trends have begun to change the very essence of the services themselves and have the potential to redefine the role of libraries.

Louise Darling stated in the last edition of the *Handbook* that

The common goal of all health science libraries is to provide access as efficiently and effectively as possible to the information resources needed in the work of the institution of which the library is a part [3].

Although access and delivery functions remain at the core of the mission of libraries, some of the basic principles are at the brink of transformation. Access to information is as important to libraries as ownership of it, and the line between in-house and external resources is blurred. The roles of the library and the individual user in information access and delivery are changing, with the direct access of users to electronic indexes, online catalogs, and document suppliers. Citation searching and document delivery services have been combined, and electronically stored text can be supplied on demand by fax or over the Internet.

Libraries find themselves in the simultaneous positions of providing traditional access and delivery services, incorporating automation to offer additional options or improvements to users, modifying services due to legal and economic considerations, and examining how services and the role of libraries themselves should evolve.

Economic trends have influenced access and delivery services to an ever increasing extent. The decline in the purchasing power of library acquisitions budgets and shrinking institutional financial resources have increased the importance of meeting informational needs through external sources. As the introduction to the revision of the "National Interlibrary Loan Code" points out, changes in the last decade have made interlibrary cooperation an integral element of collection development for libraries, rather than an ancillary option to building a local collection [4]. Economic constraints have also accelerated the desire to take advantage of electronic access to information. The identification of costs and comparative benefits, appropriate fees and charges, and fee-based services has become critical to the management of access and delivery services.

The Association of Research Libraries finds that these factors have caused the current interlibrary loan system in academic libraries to reach the breaking point [5]. It calls for reexamination and redesign of the system, including rethinking of local processes, substitution of user-initiated activity for current staff and paper functions, integration of alternative suppliers into the interlibrary loan stream, and innovative uses of technology [6].

Legal considerations also require more attention. The application of the copyright law to access and delivery services changes as there are new legal decisions, new technologies, and services which are new, are offered to new user groups, or are fee-based. The Americans with Disabilities Act is also important legislation for libraries to consider in determining how access and delivery services are provided.

Health sciences libraries are faced with a number of challenges in access and delivery: to develop effective organizational models to manage these services, to make choices about technology and to implement systems, to recover costs and generate sources of funding, and to determine and assume new roles.

In spite of the impact of technology, the importance of the human element in access and delivery services remains constant. An American Library Association manual published in 1919 noted that:

> Successful loan work calls for distinctly human qualities rather than a scholar's equipment or technical training. It is the point of immediate and constant contact between the library and its public, and makes or breaks the library's reputation for service and courtesy [7].

With the exception of the requirement of technical training for staff, the statement is still a fair assessment of the importance of access and delivery services and the critical role of staff.

Organization of Volume

Information Access and Delivery in Health Sciences Libraries is organized so that the whole volume or individual chapters may be read as needed. Readers interested in specific types of services may wish to consult relevant portions of the first chapter on administration and organization and the last chapter on recent advances and future trends, as well as the chapter on the particular service.

Chapter 1, by Susan Russell Lessick, covers administration and organization for all access and delivery services, including the organizational framework, budgeting, staffing and training, policies, and performance measures. The impact of the copyright law on all access and delivery services is reviewed in depth here; this section pulls together valuable information and current analysis from a variety of sources. The author stresses the implications of increased emphasis on access to information and on user-centered services.

The subject of Chapter 2 is circulation services and physical access to local resources. Valerie L. Su discusses the effect on access of collection arrangement, circulation systems, self-service photocopying, services for persons with disabilities, stacks maintenance, security, and building considerations. The continuing importance of hands-on access to collection resources, and how to facilitate it, underlies the information presented.

In Chapter 3, Gretchen Naisawald Arnold and Martha R. Fishel look at trends and operations and procedures for interlibrary borrowing and lending and document delivery, the development of technology-based systems, and current options for automated interlibrary loan and document delivery. The impact of technology is clearly evident by the expanded coverage of the topic in the chapter. In the most recent edition of the *Handbook*, automated interlibrary loan systems were anticipated, but actual practice was largely limited to the use of automated systems for verifying citations and identifying locations and to the use of the OCLC ILL subsystem or electronic mail for sending requests for materials. DOCLINE was in an experimental stage, and fax was not yet deemed practical for general use in transmitting documents [8]. The advances in technology and the staggering array of options for acquiring documents today are examined at length in this chapter.

Chapter 4 examines a new topic for the *Handbook/Current Practice* series, fee-based services. James Curtis and N.J. Wolfe define fee-based services as services or products for which a library has an established fee structure designed to recover more than direct out-of-pocket costs, and which are intended for defined user groups. The chapter traces the development of fee-based services and discusses planning, operating, and marketing fee-based access and delivery services. The authors survey the range of issues involved in these services: ethical, economic, legal, and organizational.

Chapter 5, by Beryl Glitz and Irene Lovas, concludes by observing recent advances and future trends in traditional and remote access and delivery for local and external resources and in electronic delivery, as well as the implications of the virtual library. The technological advances described not only improve the speed and variety of options of information delivery; they can change the very nature of the information delivered. The authors consider the implications for library operations and the shift in traditional library roles and copyright needs, among other issues.

Acknowledgments

Many people volunteered their time and the benefit of their experience to this volume. The editor is grateful to Alison Bunting, Editor-in-Chief of *Current Practice in Health Sciences Librarianship,* for her knowledge of health sciences libraries, her wise and ever practical suggestions, and her patience and encouragement. The authors devoted much of their lives to the volume during the research and writing, and they persevered through several drafts. Their expertise and perspective are evident in the results. The volume was improved by the critical comments of the expert reviewers, who are noted following the preface, and by the legal counsel of Robert A.

Wynbrandt in the review of the copyright section. Michael Homan's assistance as MLA Managing Editor of Books has been invaluable in all phases of review and production of the volume.

Carolyn E. Lipscomb
Durham, NC

References

1. Bunting A. From Index Catalogue to gopher space: changes in our profession as reflected in the Handbook and CPHSL. Bull Med Libr Assoc 1994 Jan;82(1):1-11.

2. Ibid., 9.

3. Darling L. Public services in health science libraries: overview. In: Darling L, Bishop D, Colaianni LA, eds. Handbook of medical library practice. 4th ed. v.1. Chicago: Medical Library Association, 1982:1-13.

4. National interlibrary loan code for the United States, 1993. RQ 1994 Summer;33(4):477-9.

5. Baker SK, Jackson ME. Maximizing access, minimizing cost: a first step toward the information access future. rev. Washington, DC: Association of Research Libraries, 1993.

6. Ibid., 4.

7. Vitz CPP. Loan work. 2d ed. rev. Chicago: American Library Association, 1919. (A.L.A. manual of library economy).

8. Middleton D. Lending services: interlibrary loan/document delivery. In: Darling L, Bishop D, Colaianni LA, eds. Handbook of medical library practice. 4th ed. v.1. Chicago: Medical Library Association, 1982:95-136.

1

Administration and Organization of Services

Susan Russell Lessick

The orientation of today's libraries is shifting from collection growth to providing information access for users. It has been suggested that the change in emphasis from ownership to access can be attributed to at least two factors: "the decline in funds available to purchase materials and the effects of technological changes, which have expanded accessibility to users without requiring ownership by the user's primary library" [1]. Understanding and evaluating accessibility along with other long-range fiscal and technological changes, therefore, have become essential to designing effective contemporary information services, including library services such as circulation, interlibrary loan, and fee-based services. It is equally critical to understand this development in order to establish and enhance the organization and management structures that support those services.

The growing importance of information access and delivery functions in health sciences libraries places an increased emphasis on the information user [2]. This "client-centered" view of library services presents both a challenge and an opportunity for library planners in terms of the nature and types of services offered and library operations in general. The new emphasis on access issues requires what has been called "a holistic view of the information user" [3], or viewing operations from an integrated approach. Rather than thinking of library operations in strictly conventional terms of public and technical divisions, access services presupposes increased interaction between functions, and even a convergence of functions, to obtain the greater goal of providing access to the world of information.

The new emphasis has impelled several management trends, including the creation of new alignments of functions such as the development of access services departments and the increased integration of traditional divisions within a library. This focus on access, in combination with other factors, has created a larger service role for circulation in ensuring quality library service and user satisfaction. Interlibrary loan services have come to the forefront of library activities, as libraries increasingly need to obtain external materials through resource sharing and by other commercial means. Evolving access policies increasingly reflect a user-centered focus while balancing financial and legal considerations. The renewed interest in the effectiveness of user access to information resources and the growing demand for accountability have prompted more and more libraries to use measurements to improve the management of library services.

This chapter describes the recent organizational shift from circulation to access services and the expanded integration of library functions. It describes the organizational framework of the two largest units that comprise access services, circulation and interlibrary loan, and highlights the areas of staffing, training, and policies for these areas. This chapter also explores a number of other important issues and challenges characteristic of managing circulation and interlibrary loan, including the growing use of performance measures to better understand and evaluate access services and the copyright implications of access services, broken down by various types of activities.

Toward an Access Services Organizational Model

Steel has observed that one of the more conspicuous organizational trends in U.S. libraries in the past decade has been the creation of a department or division known as "access services" [4]. This trend can also be observed in larger health sciences libraries, which have either restructured the alignment of units or renamed existing units to reflect the newer, integrated approach to access and delivery functions. A survey conducted using the MEDLIB-L list server indicated that seven academic libraries had recently instituted, or were seriously considering establishing, access services divisions within their libraries [5]. These relatively new and still evolving departments are responsible for the services and operations that enable users to locate, obtain, and efficiently use health sciences information without regard to format, function, and location. A 1991 survey of large academic libraries showed an extremely wide variation of functions falling under the umbrella of access services, including most public service functions, except reference, as well as traditional technical services functions such as bindery and preservation, although these arrangements were rare. The survey also indicated that the number of functions currently ascribed to access services is growing [6].

Circulation is the core responsibility of, and the function most usually associated with, the access services model. Other functions commonly assigned to access services include stack maintenance, reserves, billing, and library security [7]. Surveys indicate that interlibrary loan is also frequently incorporated within access services [8-9]. Other areas assigned to access services in health sciences libraries were media and photocopy services [10].

That access services departments will continue to develop gradually within library organizations is evident both by the diversity of functions that fall within them and by the fact that these departments continue to incorporate additional functional responsibilities. The growing prevalence of this organizational model seems to indicate that it has a great deal of flexibility and has the potential for meeting the needs of a variety of library organizations while at the same time meeting the needs of the information user.

Increased Integration of Traditional Functions

While there appears to be growing recognition that in the future new alignments of access functions may be necessary to enhance the user's information access, long-standing library structures with compartmental-ized divisions and work units, which have traditionally supported access and delivery services, are still largely in place. However, even in tradition-ally managed libraries there is a growing trend to moderate the divisional or compartmentalized structure and better integrate all library functions and units. Many libraries make extensive use of committees and task forces which cross departmental or divisional lines. Also, split assignments, cross staffing, and cross training are commonly used to bring divisions and units closer to each other and to the user. The growing use of matrix management techniques in libraries also promotes more effective coordination and inte-gration of functions.

Coordination among various access services units is vital in maximizing resources, sharing expertise, and improving the services of each. Strong relationships exist among circulation, cataloging, and collection develop-ment units. Interlibrary loan maintains productive and important linkages with reference, collection development, and cataloging. Substantial coordi-nation and communication between interrelated units enhances the units involved and consequently enhances services to the user. These important interrelationships are explored in detail in discussions of circulation and interlibrary loan services later in the chapter.

Circulation: The Core of Access Services

As a result of evolving library interests, management trends, and the introduction of automated systems, the role, scope, and contribution of circulation services in academic libraries have greatly fluctuated over the years. Carver has traced the three major organizational shifts of circulation from the turn of the century to present day [11]. Until World War II circulation played a broad, central, and highly visible role that reflected the collection-focused interests of the library profession at that time. The unit's scope narrowed drastically after the war, however, and was reduced to highly mechanized book-charging activities, being staffed primarily by clerical assistants. Carver argues this was the result of implementing scientific management theory which emphasized the micro-management concepts of specialization, division of labor, and increased efficiency [12].

Since the early 1980s, however, circulation's role has expanded once again. Carver suggests that the growing prevalence of the new access services structure is an evolutionary outgrowth of circulation services taking on a broader purpose and larger service role [13]. Presently circulation is an essential, complex, and interactive public-centered access unit which makes numerous broad organizational contributions to other library units, such as catalog maintenance and collection development. Through convenient and effective systems, efficient and integrated practices, and user policies that maximize the use of the collection, well-managed circulation services are essential in ensuring the quality of access services and will determine to a large extent the user's ability to successfully locate, obtain, and use library resources.

Organizational Considerations

Whether circulation is structurally related to other access and delivery units such as interlibrary loan (ILL) or is a stand-alone department, circulation functions usually incorporate certain standard responsibilities. In larger health sciences libraries these circulation responsibilities have historically merged circulation desk, stacks maintenance, and collection security functions. Routine desk functions include discharging materials to users, renewing materials, checking materials' status, handling library card applications, and placing holds and recalls. Other important frontline functions, undervalued in the past, include assisting clients in locating materials and providing basic information and reference assistance. These latter functions are especially important during night and weekend hours when the reference desk is not staffed.

The circulation unit is also responsible for various essential processing tasks that are performed behind the scenes. These processing tasks must be done with diligence and consistency. They include searching for missing materials; replacing or withdrawing missing materials; processing library cards, overdues, holds, and recalls; and billing for replacements. The circulation unit is also responsible for performing administrative duties such as reporting and analyzing statistics, scheduling desk hours and meetings, and training staff.

The circulation desk staff also commonly handles stacks maintenance, which normally entails systematic materials pickup within the library, date-stamping materials used within the library, sorting materials to be reshelved, reshelving materials, and straightening stacks. Other stacks maintenance duties include shelf reading, shifts, and collection inventories. The circulation staff also monitors the exit control gate for collection security.

Some libraries group together other closely related services such as reserves, photocopy, current periodicals, media, and microforms. These groupings vary depending on the size, type, and physical organization of the library.

The organizational structure of circulation depends primarily on the size and use of the library's collection and the overall governance structure of library. In small libraries with one person, circulation functions are fully integrated into other library activities. Larger libraries compartmentalize functions and assign certain duties to professional staff and others to the support staff or to student assistants. Usually circulation units in large health sciences libraries are structured along functional lines. Circulation and access services units are commonly placed within the public services division. Reporting lines for both are normally to the head or administrator of public services.

Circulation must particularly interact and cooperate with two other functional divisions in the library: cataloging and collection development. Out of necessity and as a result of the sophistication of integrated library systems, circulation now plays an active role in database maintenance, both in helping to create and to maintain the bibliographic database. Its relationship with collection development also requires meaningful communication and coordination. Inventory control systems and resource use studies, administered by circulation/access services, provide a wealth of statistical detail; anecdotal reports on building traffic, user problems, and the like, tracked by circulation/access services, provide critical information for resource selection decisions and collection management.

Budgeting and Fund Management

Circulation budgeting practices vary among health sciences libraries and are determined by the functions assigned to circulation and the existing budgeting allocation system of the parent institution. Major budgetary components for circulation include personnel, internal operating expenses, and equipment. The principal budgetary outlay for circulation is for salaries that support the base staffing level needed to carry out circulation tasks such as loan desk, overdues, billing, withdrawing materials, shelving, and other related tasks. Operating expenses include costs for forms such as registration and overdues notices, date due slips, date bands and stamps, book pockets and cards if used, book trucks, printing expenditures, postage, and security system supplies such as magnetized book detection strips and bar-coded labels. Other operating expenditures include service agreement costs associated with maintaining equipment, security, and automated systems. If the circulation function generates revenue through fines, cost recovery expenses for billing and collection agency fees are included in the budget. Capital expenditures may also be necessary and vary depending on the presence of automated security and circulation systems, the type and number of systems employed, and whether the automated circulation system is part of a larger library automation program.

If circulation services generate income from library access fees or in some cases coin-operated photocopy machines, cash control records and cash handling procedures should be established at the circulation desk. In cases where libraries levy fines for overdues and to recover lost book costs, the circulation staff need to prepare and send bills to users for unreturned library materials. Costs frequently included in the billing process are the cost of the material and any processing costs that may have been incurred in the notification and replacement process. Usually the fiscal structure of the library or institution permits funds realized from overdues and lost book fines to be used for replacement items. Fund management practices at the circulation desk should be in conformity with generally accepted accounting principles, institutional practices, and other applicable regulatory procedures. For efficiency, circulation billing activities should be coordinated with billing units of the parent institution.

Staffing

Determining the nature and appropriate level of personnel support needed to staff a circulation desk depends on a number of organizational and environmental factors. Jones and Kasses cite the following important determinants: collection size and usage, average number of users, and number of hours the library is open [14]. Additional factors that play a significant role in formulating staffing practices concern the variety of functions that take place at the desk, the need for backup support, and the use of automated circulation systems, including self-service check-out systems.

Jones and Kasses also describe how size affects circulation staffing and suggest that as a library grows, its circulation staff becomes increasingly more specialized with certain duties assigned to various categories of personnel [15]. They point out that in one-person libraries, all functions are performed by a single individual. In larger libraries with one professional librarian and several support staff, the support staff generally cover the circulation desk while the professional oversees library operations and services. Large health sciences libraries, on the other hand, have numerous support staff and student assistants to handle the volume and diversity of circulation work. In these libraries it is also customary to have a full-time head of circulation or supervisor to oversee activities. This staff member may either be highly skilled support staff or a professional librarian.

The need for a full-time librarian to oversee circulation activities has been the subject of debate among professionals. It has been suggested that professional staffing of the circulation unit is justified in that this frontline function is crucial to the overall success of the library [16]. Since circulation personnel are the principal agents in projecting a competent image to library users, libraries would be best served if the "image agent" were a service-oriented professional trained to anticipate the needs and problems of users. Whatever category of staff person is assigned to supervise circulation activities, however, it should be recognized that this staff member plays a critical role in promoting both the library's image and the user's satisfaction.

Night and weekend supervision of the library is of constant concern to libraries. Smaller hospital libraries with limited staff support usually maintain normal business hours and provide various mechanisms for after-hours access. These include calling a security guard, using a magnetic card reader, keypad doorknob, or video camera at the library door, or leaving a key in another open area in the hospital for sign-out [17]. Volunteers will oftentimes staff the small hospital library if hours are actually extended. Larger libraries employ either support staff or experienced student assistants to staff the library at these times. Whatever the situation, individuals assigned night and weekend supervision responsibilities should be dependable and have good judgment as they are responsible for the operation of the entire library.

Circulation staff of large libraries frequently perform functions usually associated with other library units. This common practice is an efficient way to assist overburdened units while keeping the circulation staff busy during slow desk times, such as nights and weekends. Circulation staff may assist by providing reference service during evenings and weekends [18], with various interlibrary loan billing and clerical functions, as well as assisting with tasks such as addressing and packaging ILL materials. Due to staff reductions and coverage problems, an increasing number of libraries are cross training and using staff in creative and untraditional ways to ensure that critical functions are maintained effectively and efficiently.

Student assistants are often employed by large academic libraries because they provide a readily available, inexpensive work force. They are willing to perform very routine functions, such as shelving and stacks maintenance, and are flexible about the unique scheduling needs of a library. Students are frequently used to cover peak periods of library activity related to the academic cycle and to cover nights and weekends and other difficult to staff hours. They are particularly useful as backups for individuals on vacation or sick leave and in meeting special project needs. While many staff coverage problems can be eliminated through the use of student assistants, supervisors should be cautioned that student employment poses a number of supervisory challenges. Common personnel problems associated with student employment include high turnover rates, sudden and inconvenient terminations, school or work scheduling conflicts, and examination period absenteeism.

Because professional and graduate students are often unavailable for part-time work, the recruitment and retention of student assistants in academic health sciences libraries can be difficult. This situation is exacerbated if the health sciences campus or branch is separated from the university campus. In these cases health sciences libraries may have to draw student assistants from other area institutions or hire library support staff in lower personnel classifications to fill critical positions and to ensure essential functions are consistently and effectively carried out.

Volunteers are another important category of personnel often present in circulation units. This is particularly true in hospital libraries. Volunteers may be useful in performing a variety of circulation and processing tasks. Special care, however, should be taken in scheduling volunteers and assigning them tasks, as meeting the needs of both the volunteer and the library can sometimes be difficult.

The circulation staff is one of the most important elements in the successful achievement of a library's service mission. Studies have shown that the circulation staff is the user's primary contact within the library and that the user judges the quality of the library and services it provides based on initial contact with the circulation unit [19]. A well-trained and service-oriented circulation staff is essential in assuring that the user's problems and needs are quickly identified and user satisfaction is guaranteed.

Training

The circulation staff has an impact upon everyone who comes to the library. For this reason, it is almost impossible to overemphasize the importance of well-trained and friendly circulation staff. Effective training and development programs for circulation staff vary from library to library, but there are some basic training tools and methods that are useful in training the members of any size circulation staff.

Most successful circulation training programs include written training manuals, handouts, or training checklists. A procedure or operating manual may be substituted for a training manual if the procedures are up to date, detailed, complete, and clear. The manual is an essential guide to training staff and should provide methods of handling both routine procedures and unusual problems. It should be placed in a strategic location and used as a reference after training is complete. Training should also include practical on-site demonstrations as well as actual experience monitored closely at first by a supervisor. Training may also be supplemented by audiovisual and computer-assisted instruction (CAI) materials. If circulation tasks include using specific types of computer programs, new personnel can use hands-on tutorials which may accompany the programs. Using advanced learning technologies may improve training programs in two ways: first, they permit new employees to use the materials independently and at their own pace; and second, they relieve the supervisor or other staff from time-consuming individualized instruction.

Training programs for circulation staff members should consist of an overview of library operations that includes library hours; typical inquiries and referral practices; and procedures for opening and closing the library, statistical record keeping, circulation and stacks maintenance, and using automated systems. Staff should receive training in how to report mechanical, technical, and security problems and how to deal with emergencies including medical emergencies and evacuations. Training programs should also emphasize the need to treat the user courteously. If possible, staff members should attend special training sessions focusing on behaviors essential to providing positive, helpful, and friendly service. The sessions should cover problem-based situations such as doctors in a hurry or in their scrubs who have forgotten their library cards. They should also describe conflict resolution techniques and how to cope competently and courteously with "difficult" users. Training methods should also cover the interactions that take place with culturally diverse users.

An important component of circulation training involves ongoing staff development. Circulation staff training is a process that requires continual attention and does not end after the initial training period. Additional training may be necessary if employees still lack certain skills; if policies, procedures, and equipment are altered; or if new services require new knowledge or skills. Written handouts announcing new services, materials, and procedural changes are essential for this purpose and should be continued after the initial training period. Refresher courses may also be useful in maintaining good technical and interpersonal performance. A diverse work force presents both opportunities and challenges for the library supervisor or trainer. Typically, personnel hired to work in the library come from a wide variety of backgrounds and cultures. This diversity poses some interesting problems for the trainer who must understand that varied cultural values and practices produce varied learning styles. Diverse learning activities should contribute to the effectiveness of the training program in reaching all staff members.

Collection Access Policies

User access policies and practices for resources and services are the very foundation of library services and operations. Access policies relate to in-library and external use of collections, to information services such as reference, and to other facilities matters such as regulations on study facilities, copying equipment, and prohibitions on eating and smoking except in designated areas. The following discussion applies primarily to collection access, specifically lending policies. Well-considered and clear lending policies allow for the equitable distribution of library resources [20] and should incorporate an "access philosophy" or user-centered focus whenever possible. Access services personnel play an important role in policy formation, application, and communication because of their high degree of direct contact with users and their knowledge of user needs and problems [21]. Access policies vary depending on many factors such as the category of user, the unit's goals and objectives, and the format and function of library materials. In addition, lending policies are shaped increasingly by budgetary, technological, ethical, and legal considerations.

Lending Policies

User Considerations

Determinations about who will use the library's services and resources are critical and fundamental policy decisions all health sciences libraries must make. The establishment of user policies in both large and small health sciences libraries is a collaborative effort among the library, its primary users, and appropriate administrative authorities. In developing user policies, the library must first identify and categorize various user groups, then determine primary and secondary users, and then finally decide which policies should apply to which group. Policies must be clearly delineated, without regard to the simplicity or complexity of the resulting document. The final policy document should be stored in an access or operation manual that is readily available to library personnel. In addition, access policy handouts, pamphlets, and brochures should be available to library users, and access policy statements should be visible at the library's entrance. By ensuring the uniform application of access policies, user policy documents are helpful to library personnel and library users alike. Topper maintains that user policies should reflect and advance the goals of the parent institution [22]. In academic and large hospital libraries with strong teaching commitments, user policies should provide active library support for faculty, residents, and students. Hospital libraries with primarily clinical and patient care missions should provide extensive access privileges to the hospital's medical staff and other members of the patient care team.

In academic libraries, primary users are usually defined as students, faculty, and staff. Many academic libraries assign different privileges to various segments of the primary user population. For example, faculty members may be extended more generous borrowing privileges than are students or staff members, and graduate students may be granted different privileges than undergraduate students. Depending upon institutional and community relations policies, the public may or may not be allowed collection access privileges.

A hospital library's primary user group usually includes the hospital's medical staff; the hospital's general employee population; students, if it is a teaching hospital; and designated affiliated users if cooperative agreements exist. Primary users in hospital libraries may or may not be further subdivided depending on a variety of factors.

It is generally advisable to limit the number of primary user privileges, so that that they are easy for users to understand and for library staff to apply. This limitation may not always be possible, however, given the various educational, clinical, and research cultures within which libraries exist, and in light of various technological and economic changes currently affecting libraries.

Increasingly health sciences libraries are establishing user policies that extend access privileges to patients and their families. The standards for hospital libraries of both the Joint Commission on Accreditation of Healthcare Organizations (JCAHO) [23] and the Medical Library Association (MLA) [24] require that libraries make their resources accessible for patient education and participate with other hospital departments and services to coordinate hospital-wide patient education efforts. These developments are due in large measure to changing attitudes toward health consumer's rights and a recognition that informed patients facilitate the maintenance of personal health and quality patient care decisions. According to a recent survey of health sciences libraries, a large majority of hospital and academic libraries provide some form of access to facilities, resources, and services by patients [25]. Patient access policies should describe the goals and extent of services provided, the relationship of the library to other institutional patient education programs, and the referral practices to relevant institutional and community resources. MLA's recently adopted "A Code of Ethics for Health Sciences Librarianship" states that health sciences librarians should "promote access to health information for all" [26]. Libraries should make some provision for extending access to library facilities, collections, and services to patients and their families directly or by actively collaborating with others to ensure that patient education and information needs are met.

User policies are also shaped by regional and national cooperative developments. For example, an academic health sciences library may be part of a larger multisite university system and participate in liberal reciprocal agreements with other institutions in the system. Large universities may extend free borrowing privileges to all faculty members of higher education institutions in their state, as is the practice at the University of California. Libraries may also establish special reciprocal agreements or affiliations with certain specialized libraries based on mutual needs and interests. Also, hospital libraries may extend access privileges to physicians and employees of other hospitals within a multihospital system. The Reciprocal Faculty Borrowing Program of the Research Libraries Advisory Committee to OCLC is an example of a national access agreement that grants library privileges to faculty members of other research universities that are Association of Research Libraries (ARL) members.

Special gratis privileges can be extended to certain designated groups such as voluntary clinical faculty in the community, institutional alumni, or friends of the library members. It is also common for academic libraries to grant lending privileges to visiting faculty, lecturers, and students from other educational institutions. Hospital libraries may give library privileges to students in affiliated educational programs, participants in continuing education courses, local health professionals, and other consortia members. Caution is recommended when extending borrowing privileges to temporary users, as only limited control can be exercised over these users; in these cases, borrowing privileges should be restricted to the duration of the user's stay.

The worsening fiscal condition of health sciences libraries in the 1980s and 1990s has had an impact on user policies. The budgetary reductions have in many cases eroded a health sciences library's ability to provide extensive access and lending privileges to secondary users. In the past, for various political, ethical, and fund development reasons, many state and federally supported health sciences libraries were hesitant about sharply curtailing the general public's access to the library and its services. An increasing number of publicly supported and private health sciences libraries, however, are limiting library access and services for external users and redirecting scant library dollars into maintaining prompt and reliable service to their primary user population. The limitations imposed upon secondary users usually include restricting the number of volumes they can check out and prohibiting them from renewing, recalling, and placing holds on materials. Some health sciences libraries restrict the access privileges of commercial information services. Some state-supported and private health sciences libraries have implemented even more drastic measures and restrict building access to primary constituents only; some libraries have found it necessary to end reciprocal borrowing agreements with other institutions entirely. And some libraries are initiating fee-based services in an attempt to recoup some of the costs of providing service to secondary users.

Loan Periods

Lending policies for library materials should provide primary users convenient access to library materials with flexible loan periods that meet the majority of their varied needs without undue restrictions and penalties. In other words, the goal of lending policies should be to provide each borrower the longest possible loan period for each item checked out without inconveniencing other borrowers. It has also been stated that lending or circulation regulations are compromises between two inconsistent library objectives: providing collection access to as many users as possible while at the same time responding effectively to individual user needs [27]. How libraries achieve this balance and realize this circulation goal differs with every library. There are as many variations of circulation regulations as there are environments in which health sciences libraries exist.

Loan periods for circulating materials vary according to the status of the borrower and the format and function of the material. Libraries generally grant primary users longer loan periods than they do secondary users. Faculty normally have longer loan periods than students, although this may be changing. Many libraries give monographs longer loan periods than they do journal issues, if they allow journal issues to circulate at all. Fragile, high-use, expensive, and rare materials generally have very short loan periods and in many cases these materials are noncirculating.

Although uniform loan periods for users and materials are easy to administer, apply, and explain, studies show that variable and shorter loan periods for heavily used materials may maximize the use of the collection and reduce user "shelf failure" and dissatisfaction. Buckland's important work on loan and duplication policies shows that user demand for books is sensitive to the availability level and that book availability can be increased by the implementation of variable loan periods on high-use items [28]. In light of these studies, the practice of extending certain users long loan periods probably should be reevaluated in an effort to increase user access and satisfaction. Whether uniform or variable loan periods are adopted, lending policies should seek a balance between what is efficient for the library and what improves user access.

Renewals, Returns, Holds, and Recalls

Lending policies for renewals and returns are intended to accommodate the need of some users for extended loan periods while ensuring the broadest use of library materials. Renewal regulations also discourage the proliferation of subcollections of library materials outside the library. Renewal regulations usually extend loan periods for users if other users have not requested or placed a hold on the material. Renewal and return regulations should stipulate whether the presentation of the materials is necessary and whether phone or e-mail renewals are permitted. Libraries usually set limits on the number of times renewals will be granted.

Increasing the availability of materials to all users is also facilitated by hold and recall policies. It is common practice in academic situations to recall materials on which reserves or holds have been placed. Hospital libraries may need to recall materials due to patient care exigencies. Most libraries set time limits on how long materials will be held for individual users before materials are reshelved or checked out by someone else. Some libraries place restrictions on the renewing, holding, and recalling of materials by secondary users.

Format Considerations

Variations in material format also affect circulation policies. Libraries usually establish different circulation regulations for monographs, journals, audiovisuals, and other formats in the collection. The 1991/92 annual statistics of the Association of Academic Health Sciences Library Directors (AAHSLD) indicate significant variations in the circulation practices of academic libraries for bound and unbound journals, monographs, and for materials in other formats [29].

Monographs. According to the AAHSLD annual statistics, monographic formats are the most likely library resources to circulate [30]. Because books take longer to read, their loan periods tend to be longer than for journals. Loan periods for monographs range from two hours to three months, depending on factors such as user demand and library setting. Some libraries set up variable loan periods for certain monographs, e.g., new books, which reflect the frequency of demand for them. More often though, variable loan periods are designated for different categories of users, as discussed earlier.

Journals. The emphasis and value that health sciences libraries place on journals has a number of implications for a library's circulation policies. Because journal materials are the very heart of health sciences libraries, and because they describe the cutting edge of scientific and medical developments, they are of critical importance to practitioners, educators, and researchers.

In light of this importance, libraries often restrict the circulation of journals, especially current issues, because of the need to increase on-site access and to ensure better control over these materials. A single journal issue usually contains numerous substantive articles, but only one or two may be of interest to the user who checks the journal out. Also, a bound volume may contain as many as a hundred articles, any or all of which may be required by other users at any given time.

Not only does journal circulation hamper access to all the articles in an issue or volume when circulating, it places the library's journal collection at risk for a variety of reasons. From a preservation point of view, circulating an unbound issue may delay the binding process, exposing the remaining issues to damage, loss, or deterioration. Bound journal volumes used outside the library are also more susceptible to loss and damage. The replacement and repair of these materials can be costly and at times impossible, a fact that is of growing concern to librarians who are faced with diminishing resources for expensive replacements. Even if monies are available, many of these materials are irreplaceable due to changes in the printing practices of many publishers.

If a library establishes a restrictive journal circulation policy, it must take other measures to make its materials available. Many libraries opt for providing an inexpensive, even free, photocopy service to eliminate the need for circulating bound and unbound journals. This service may place a heavy load on the library's photocopy equipment, but it will keep popular materials in the library for increased access. Other libraries might keep duplicate issues of heavily used journal titles and circulate them to individual borrowers and to interlibrary loan. In fact, some libraries regularly purchase two or more copies of the same journal issue in order to provide at least one circulating copy; this practice, however, is decreasing due to budgetary constraints.

If a library does not provide photocopy services or if library photocopiers are out of order, users should be allowed to remove the item from the library to use photocopy facilities elsewhere. Because of the widespread availability of photocopying equipment throughout organizations, libraries need only to permit journal circulation for very short periods. Most users can return the materials within several hours, or at the most within twenty-four hours.

It is also advisable to provide for exceptions and permit journals to circulate under certain circumstances. Many libraries with restrictive lending policies for journals still permit certain categories of serial publications such as yearbooks, annual reviews, monographic series, and conference proceedings to circulate. Other exceptions should be made if the material is needed for a classroom presentation or for slide or photographic reproduction.

Media and Microcomputer Software. Media or audiovisuals and microcomputer software programs present unique access problems for health sciences libraries. This is because the medium is fragile, is expensive when compared to paper counterparts, needs special hardware and facilities, and is relatively scarce in most libraries. Media functions principally as a teaching aid, whether in degree programs, in-service training programs, or continuing education courses. Public access microcomputer programs fulfill a variety of user needs, including patient care, education, research, and work-related needs. All of these materials, despite their special handling requirements, must be easily accessible to the library's primary users. In managing media and software, as with other library materials, libraries should be guided by the local environment, institutional requirements, and common sense.

Circulation for most nonbook materials is usually restricted to on-site use by the primary library users. A growing number of libraries, however, are making an effort to facilitate their circulation outside the library and through interlibrary loan. This is especially true of audiocassettes and one-half inch videocassettes, as listening and viewing equipment is readily available in cars and homes. Another common practice is to allow instructors and departments to use these materials in the classroom. Because these materials require hardware for use, some libraries provide hardware services as well.

Because off-site use of software increases the possibility of virus contamination and because the use must be consistent with copy protection laws, electronic formats present additional access problems. These concerns result in most libraries and microcomputer centers designating software programs "library use only," though they might allow printed documentation to circulate outside the library. Technology also allows libraries to provide access to these materials via network and telecommunications connections, thus eliminating the need to circulate materials physically.

Function Considerations

Some circulation policy decisions are governed by materials characteristics, rather than user categories or format exigencies. Critically needed reference sources, highly utilized curriculum-related materials, and costly and rare items are usually housed in separate locations within the library and require special handling and access arrangements. Despite these considerations, access policies for these materials should promote their maximum use and provide on-site availability at the very least.

Reference Materials. To ensure the widest possible access by users, most health sciences libraries rarely or never circulate material in the reference collection. Basic ready reference tools such as indexes, dictionaries, and directories need to be in the library at all times. Many libraries, especially hospital libraries, prohibit circulation of key basic texts. Some libraries restrict the circulation of materials such as loose-leaf publications due to format considerations.

Reserve Materials. A reserve collection guarantees the availability of limited resources for specific groups of primary users. These groups may be students with specific reading assignments, in-service trainees, or continuing education course participants. Because libraries cannot afford to purchase enough copies to supply large educational groups, libraries are forced to limit the use of these assigned materials to short time increments. Libraries also regularly place frequently used, stolen, or damaged items on reserve.

Heavy demand reserve material usually circulates for two hours only. If certain reserve items are used less frequently, less restrictive loan periods may be applied to them, e.g., twenty-four hours, three days, or five days depending on local conditions. Regardless of how brief the circulation period, some provision for overnight use should be made as well. Usually an arbitrary time is selected at the end of the day after which reserve material may be checked out for overnight use.

Special Materials. Circulation policies for historical, archival, and rare book collections are designed to provide appropriate protection for valuable and fragile material. Consequently, highly restrictive policies usually govern the circulation of these materials. Some provision, however, should be made for the scholarly access of special materials; many libraries establish a supervised reading area for that purpose. In addition to being made available for scholarly use, special materials should also be made available for exhibition.

Policies Concerning the Confidentiality of User Records

To establish management control over the collection, health sciences libraries usually maintain either manual or automated circulation records to account for the use, special handling, and locations of materials. In most cases, libraries also develop, maintain, and update user records or registration files to locate and communicate with borrowers as part of circulation procedures. An important policy consideration in the retention of transaction and user data is the user's right to privacy.

The privacy rights of library users have long been protected by professional library organizations. Both the MLA code of ethics [31] and the American Library Association (ALA) code of ethics [32] acknowledge and defend the confidentiality of the librarian-client relationship. All library records identifying the names of library users are regarded as confidential and include not only circulation records, but also records for interlibrary loan, database searching, and other personally identifiable uses of library materials, facilities, and services such as the reference interview. When feasible, libraries should consider eliminating the identification of individuals in the data structure of stored records, particularly in electronic records. Most states, as well, have laws that provide for the confidentiality of library records [33]. This legal protection either affirms protection of a user's privacy rights or exempts library records from scrutiny under state freedom of information acts.

It is important that professional librarians uphold confidentiality standards, know about legal rights and responsibilities, and create confidentiality policies that conform with ethical standards and the law. Without written policies, libraries risk civil liability or may be subjected to penalties provided in state laws in the event that confidential records are revealed. ALA recommends that library record keeping policies include policy objectives, the roles and responsibilities of the staff involved, the types of records that are protected, relevant procedures, and the circumstances under which records will be released [34]. Confidentiality policies should be incorporated into the training manuals of all departments that need user information. For detailed information on writing effective confidentiality policies, librarians should consult the ALA's *Intellectual Freedom Manual* [35].

Policy Enforcement

Because the late return of books and book loss are severe problems in libraries, effective enforcement of lending policies is of concern to all health sciences libraries. Determining the best methods to ensure compliance with library lending rules is complex and controversial. Numerous methods have been employed by libraries including the prompt sending of overdues notices; levying nominal, heavy, and graduated fines for late materials; billing users for replacement and processing costs; referring uncollected bills to credit collection agencies; suspending the lending privileges of delinquent borrowers by using the lockout features of online circulation systems; withholding campus services such as student registration, transcripts, and diplomas; using the personnel exit clearance procedures of the parent institution; and in extreme cases, taking legal action against offending users [36-37].

While the appropriateness and efficacy of various approaches have been widely debated in the library literature, most reports are anecdotal, based on philosophical beliefs and the particular institutional culture served, and only a few studies exist that actually attempt to determine statistically significant factors that lessen the probability of unreturned materials. Burgin and Hansel conducted several replicative studies of overdues in 1981 [38], 1983 [39], and 1986 [40] showing that many of the traditional overdues practices used in public libraries such as fine structures were ineffective in reducing overdues rates. While these studies did not provide clear evidence that particular strategies were consistently effective, some factors were identified as statistically significant in the overdues process. These include speedy overdues notices, sending the bill as the final notice, and restricting the borrowing privileges of users with excessive overdues. These findings were confirmed in a study of a public library system conducted by Little [41]. The use of collection agencies and the proximity of the library to the user's residence were also identified in the Little study as relevant factors [42]. It has also been suggested that external factors outside the control of librarians such as characteristics of the population served [43] and the size of the geographic area served [44] may play significant roles in reducing the rate of overdues.

Because there is surprisingly little evidence from empirical studies that can guide policy decisions, because there is conflicting opinion on how best to handle overdues, and because of the unique nature of individual libraries and the institutions and populations they serve, libraries should develop enforcement policies based on the evidence that is available, local considerations and experience, and common sense. Policies should be administered consistently and fairly to all classes of users. Common standards of service and treatment are essential in reinforcing responsible user behavior. Exceptions to policies should be clearly understood, explained simply to users, and documented in staff manuals. Policy manuals should cover the handling of complaints about overdues, bills, or books claimed returned. The manuals should indicate when problems are referred to a supervisor and when exceptions are made and require authorization. Enforcement can also be facilitated through user education; adherence to regulations is furthered by posting rules and including policy information in library publications and orientations. If necessary, libraries should use financial incentives and other compliance measures to ensure the recovery of library material and costs. Libraries must also secure support from their parent institutions to coordinate compliance efforts institution-wide and in dealing with user resentment and complaints about the punitive actions of libraries.

Interlibrary Loan: Expanded Access Through Resource Sharing

Interlibrary loan has changed greatly over the past decade, a fact that may be attributed to the advent of automation; the general decline of library resources to fund collections, services, and operations; and the de-emphasis on collection development and increased emphasis on access service development. These changes have led to the growing recognition of the value of interlibrary loan service to overall health sciences library goals and operations. Effective and efficient ILL services are now considered to be a necessity, rather than a "sidelight" or special service as in past decades [45]. Changes in ILL utilities and the use of electronic messaging systems, telefacsimile, electronic document transmission systems, and ILL management software have contributed to fundamental changes in what services ILL provides and how it provides them.

In addition, sharp increases in borrowing and lending activities due to a myriad of factors currently affect, and will continue to affect, ILL workloads. Various records show that ILL has increased significantly in academic and health sciences libraries in the recent past: ARL annual statistics show an increase of roughly 100% in median loaned and borrowed requests from 1980 to 1990 [46-47]; AAHSLD annual statistics indicate a 56% growth rate in the mean value of borrowing transactions and a 23% increase in lending requests among academic health sciences libraries in the same ten-year period [48-49]; National Library of Medicine (NLM) lending increased by 18% in this ten-year period [50-51]. The number of network requests entered into DOCLINE increased by over 190% since the system was fully implemented in 1987, though these DOCLINE figures include the increase due to additional participating libraries [52].

Because interlibrary loan is a continually growing and changing area, it will be necessary to review regularly organizational and managerial structures in order to increase efficiency and apply technology where needed. It will be equally important for health sciences libraries to adjust available resources to accommodate growth in ILL access and investigate new methods of financing these expanding services to ensure effective and reliable services. An even larger challenge for libraries may be the recent appearance of user-oriented document delivery systems via commercial document suppliers. A health sciences library's ability to provide effective, reliable, and inexpensive service may be the determining factor as to whether libraries will be eliminated in favor of extensive reliance on external commercial sources.

Organizational Considerations

The goal of ILL in most health sciences libraries continues to be the borrowing and lending of materials among libraries. Increasingly, however, libraries are using commercial document suppliers in lieu of other libraries to fill ILL requests. Common reasons for using these nontraditional sources include speed of delivery, copyright compliance, and cost. Libraries are also developing in-house document delivery services that meet client needs from their own holdings and from commercial suppliers. Another development of note is that more and more libraries are charging for ILL services. Tasks that are an integral part of contemporary interlibrary loan services include bibliographic verification; lender selection including commercial suppliers; document retrieval, photocopying, or scanning; transmission and receipt of requests via electronic ILL networks, telefacsimile, or the Internet; and the delivery of ILL requests by mail, telefacsimile, or the Internet. In addition, ILL personnel may perform various fund accounting and management tasks such as reporting and analyzing statistics.

The organization of ILL functions within libraries varies greatly and depends on such factors as the size of the collection and user community, the level of borrowing and lending activity, and the general management structure of the library. In small libraries where use is minimal, ILL functions are usually absorbed as an additional assignment by one or two staff members. As the activity level of outgoing and incoming requests grows, ILL functions are performed on a regular basis by designated staff members. In moderately sized libraries, the borrowing and lending functions are usually handled by a combination of reference and circulation staff, with the reference librarian coordinating the effort.

In larger libraries with heavy workloads, a separate ILL section with its own staff is responsible for interlibrary loan services. These ILL units may in turn be subdivided along functional lines with certain staff designated for borrowing transactions and others for lending tasks. If document delivery services are provided, tasks such as paging, photocopying, and delivering materials are usually absorbed by the ILL unit as well, although some document delivery offices function within circulation or as independent units. Larger ILL operations may also have public service counters to facilitate the consultation between the library staff and the user.

How large ILL units relate structurally to other library units depends a great deal on the local library environment and differs from library to library. Frequently, they are part of larger departments such as access/circulation services or reference services; ILL units may also be separate departmental entities. Consequently, reporting lines for interlibrary loan units vary according to where they reside within the management structure of the institution. ILL commonly reports to either the head of reference, of access/circulation, or of public services. Even in large units, functions are not entirely self-contained. ILL relies on reference for technical assistance in bibliographic verification, and the reference desk staff may even review all borrowing requests for completeness and accuracy. ILL routinely interacts with circulation in verifying the circulation status of requested items, in checking out materials needed for lending, and in securing items from processing areas. ILL also cooperates with the circulation staff by coordinating the reshelving of pulled ILL materials with other library materials. If photocopying and billing are handled by a section other than ILL, the ILL section must work closely with that section as well. In addition, the ILL staff is in a position to provide information to technical services on completeness and accuracy of bibliographic records and other operations which can lead to improvements in other library services.

The role of interlibrary loan in collection development is the subject of much discussion in the professional literature [53]. It is usually assumed that the titles most frequently requested for interlibrary loan are the titles that should be considered for first purchase. In many cases, however, this may not be an accurate assessment as frequently requested materials may be of individualized interest and fall outside the scope of the library's collection. Frequency counts of requested titles are insufficient in and of themselves in identifying potential serial and monographic titles for purchase; but considered with other important factors, they can be important tools in identifying the user's information needs and the collection's weaknesses. Interlibrary loan can also improve user access to materials by reporting missing titles and pages to collection development personnel so that replacement action can be taken.

Budgeting, Costs, and Charges

The development of an operating budget for interlibrary loan depends largely on the overall budgeting structure of the library or parent institution and the amount of revenue generated by the service itself. Smaller net-borrowing libraries or libraries that have reciprocal borrowing agreements with other institutions use expense summaries to detail costs; in these cases the library fully absorbs all expenses related to ILL. Larger health sciences libraries which are net lenders and generate substantial amounts of income frequently track ILL expenditures and income, offset expenditures with income, and determine final net income, using an accounts receivable/payable structure that is part of a larger institutional fund accounting system. The resulting revolving accounts are budgeted annually and usually have a "fall back" account that can be debited should a negative balance occur in the primary account.

The three most important budget categories for ILL are personnel, operational supplies and services, and equipment. Salaries for staff, including professionals, paraprofessionals, clerks, and students, are by far the single largest budgetary expense for the ILL unit. Any necessary training expenditures for staff should also be reflected in the budget. Internal operating expenses include consumable supplies, network and communication costs, utilities such as DOCLINE and OCLC, online database costs related to bibliographic searching and verification, photocopy and fax costs, and routine and expedited delivery costs. Externally imposed borrowing expenses include loan charges, copyright royalty charges, routine and expedited delivery charges, fax charges, and charges from commercial document suppliers. If the lending operation generates significant revenue, cost recovery expenses such as billing, recharging, and purchased coupons expenses should also be considered. Expenditures for capital equipment, such as upgrading and replacing hardware and software, maintaining equipment, and renewing rental agreements, can also be a sizable expense.

Having cost data and understanding the economics of interlibrary loan are of great interest to all libraries. To the extent that a library functions as a lender, detailed cost studies allow for more accurate lending fees to be established, either at full or partial cost recovery. Understanding ILL costs is important for preparing and forecasting budgets, for analyzing work flow for greater efficiency, for selecting potential lenders, for comparing traditional ILL lenders with nontraditional lenders, for making informed collection development decisions about buying or borrowing specific titles, and for convincing funding bodies of the value of ILL [54].

Various methods and tools are available to determine actual ILL costs accurately [55]. In general, the most accurate costs include all direct costs incurred by the borrower or lender and include both filled and unfilled requests [56]. Indirect administrative overhead costs, or costs that would be incurred whether or not a library participated in ILL, are generally excluded. The conventional unit most commonly used by health sciences libraries in assessing the costs of ILL is the average (mean) cost per filled request at the lending agency. Using this methodology, NLM and the Regional Medical Libraries regularly conduct cost studies of filled, referred, and rejected ILL requests to establish the national maximum charge for the National Network of Libraries of Medicine (NN/LM).

Other important studies have been conducted with varying results depending on the methodology used to define and categorize costs. Through a joint ILL survey project sponsored by both the Research Libraries Group (RLG) and ARL, efforts to standardize categories of included and excluded ILL costs and to create one uniform cost model were recently undertaken among research libraries. Results from this large benchmark study show that the cost of one completed ILL transaction (borrowing and lending libraries' cost combined) averages $29.55; this breaks down as $18.62 for one filled borrowing transaction and $10.93 for one filled lending transaction [57]. Additional efforts are needed in analyzing cost differences among libraries and in further standardizing methodologies for determining costs. The development of a uniform cost model for ILL units in all types of libraries would allow more meaningful comparisons and conclusions to be drawn and help identify the most cost-effective procedures.

Unlike their university and public library counterparts, health sciences libraries have shown a sustained interest in ILL cost recovery for quite some time [58]. Arcari attributes this early interest in cost recovery to several factors, including the practices and policies of NLM and National Institutes of Health (NIH) and the financial structure of academic health centers themselves [59]. These underlying factors, in conjunction with the widespread need to generate funds for additional staffing and equipment, have resulted in health sciences libraries shifting from wholly subsidized ILL services to a fee-for-service model, wherein the user bears the financial burden of the service.

ILL charges fall into two categories: borrowing and lending charges. Ordinarily the internal costs of processing borrowing requests, whether known or unknown, are automatically absorbed by the borrowing library, though some libraries have begun to assess a flat transaction fee to process borrowing requests. These fees are normally used to cover some or all of the charges levied against the borrowing institution by the lending institution. Libraries which do not assess a processing fee either absorb or pass on to the end user any ILL borrowing charges incurred. Some libraries set aside a portion of their acquisitions budget for ILL borrowing charges on the principle that when access is provided in lieu of ownership the cost of access should be supported by the library.

Of concern to health sciences libraries, and other libraries as well, are lending charges levied on external institutions for supplying a loan request. Most of the discussion in the literature concerns ILL lending charges and how best to determine what these charges should be. ILL lending charges differ from library to library depending on a wide variety of factors, including the cost setting policy and service philosophy of the library,

library-specific costs, the fiscal and procedural requirements of the parent institution, network fees, and the fee systems of Resource Libraries, Regional Medical Libraries, and NLM. In 1994 the maximum amount charged by Resource and Regional Medical Libraries was $10.00, although not all libraries charge the maximum fee. Beginning in 1992, NLM charged $8.00 for each filled domestic request, $10.00 for a foreign loan, and a $3.00 surcharge for material sent by telefacsimile.

Staffing

The level and type of staff needed for interlibrary loan services depend primarily on the extent of borrowing and lending activity of the library. Smaller library operations may divide the workload among several staff members, usually between a professional and the circulation support staff. In these work situations, the professional assumes the supervisory and bibliographic verification functions, and the support staff carries out various clerical, transmission, paging, photocopying, and mailing functions. Professional participation in ILL activities and a similar division of tasks are also commonplace in larger academic and health sciences libraries, though these libraries also use student assistants for lower level tasks. Larger libraries are increasingly using highly knowledgeable and skilled support staff to perform many tasks such as bibliographic searching, online transmission and receipt of requests, and various records management functions. In these situations professionals assist by resolving complex verification and location problems, interpreting policy and rules if necessary, and directing operations. Professional input in ILL has been shown to have a measurable impact on the quality of service [60], and thus it continues to play an important role in ensuring effective ILL services.

Because of their complexity, borrowing requests require a higher proportion of professional participation than do lending requests. A large portion of lending tasks do not require highly paid or highly trained staff, since these tasks involve paging, photocopying, scanning, wrapping, and mailing materials. Consequently, it is common for lower level support staff, student assistants, and, in the case of hospital libraries, volunteers, to perform effectively the majority of lending functions. Because borrowing requests are considerably more complicated, borrowing functions are the most time-consuming to complete. Studies of large academic libraries show that processing borrowing requests requires about 2.5 times as much staff time as processing lending requests [61], although this may apply less to health sciences libraries, where borrowing focuses on current material and consequently is more straightforward than it might be in an academic library.

When ILL demand is high and a sizable unexpected increase in requests ensues, temporary assistance may be needed to supplement existing staff. During peak operating periods, ILL staff will often move back and forth between lending and borrowing functions. In addressing staff shortages in lending, however, care should be taken not to cross staff to the point that borrowing effectiveness is inadvertently diminished and ILL service quality as a whole suffers. Assistance may be necessary from circulation or reference staff members in reducing any backlog; it may also be possible to transfer some of the workload to another cooperating library. Access departments and library organizations should prepare beforehand through planning and cross training so that they can shift staff quickly and react to warning signs of overload or bottlenecks at the earliest opportunity. A flexible and responsive staffing approach to ILL, as well as other operations, ensures that quality and efficient services, even at extremely busy times, are maintained.

A growing management concern is the need for adequate staffing to cope with the increasing demand for ILL services and how best to justify those needs. Various measures are used to help demonstrate that a particular library has an unreasonable workload and therefore requires more staff. Some of these indicators include output (requests processed/FTE), fill rate (requests filled/requested), turnaround time, and user satisfaction. Measurement tools, such as the self-analysis work form of the ARL Office of Management Studies [62], are available to facilitate workload analysis. Using these tools, along with an analytical examination process, may reveal strengths or weaknesses in ILL operations, and the results may serve as a viable argument in justifying the need for increased staffing or other desired changes.

With the increased emphasis on interlibrary loan service and resource sharing in libraries, a highly effective and efficient ILL staff has become essential to the overall success of the library. Smaller collection budgets and new technology have significantly increased the workloads and have changed methods of operation of ILL units. A highly skilled, organized, intuitive, and motivated ILL staff is indispensable in coping with the pressure of heavy workloads and a rapidly changing work environment.

Training

The ILL staff is the critical link between the local library user and the outside world of information. Effective training of personnel is of paramount importance because the quality and efficiency of ILL service depend on how well and how quickly they do their work. With the advent of new technologies, requisite knowledge and skills of ILL personnel have changed and increased over the past decade. In addition to knowing internal procedures, reference tools and catalogs, local, state and national lending codes, and copyright law, the ILL staff must now be competent in various complex systems and technologies. These include the use of internal and remote online catalogs such as the Locator, NLM's online public catalog accessible through the Internet; CD-ROM systems; MEDLINE and other bibliographic databases; ILL utilities such as DOCLINE, OCLC, and the Ariel document transmission system; commercial document delivery systems; telefacsimile; Internet; and a variety of other software systems related to telecommunications and record maintenance. Borrowing unit personnel, in particular, need substantial bibliographic expertise and computer skills.

Although training of ILL staff should be geared to local and regional needs, some general guidelines apply in almost all situations. As in other library departments, ILL training should include a general orientation, demonstrations, hands-on experience, the initial checking of work, and the use of audiovisuals and software if appropriate and available. In addition, ongoing staff development is important to ensure that ILL personnel keep informed of emerging technologies.

All libraries should have a well-written, up-to-date training or operating manual of internal interlibrary loan procedures and policies which describes in a step-by-step manner instructions for various ILL procedures. The manual can also provide guidance to others outside the unit when providing backup due to illness or vacations. Actual training manuals or tutorial sections of user manuals for various ILL utilities are available in the NLM *DOCLINE Manual* [63] and the *OCLC Workbook: Using the PRISM Service* [64]. These are essential training tools for new staff and help them learn the log-on/log-off, transmit/receive, and status checking procedures of commonly used ILL systems. General user manuals of DOCLINE, Loansome Doc, PRISM, and Ariel systems are excellent references for both novice and experienced users.

Training in the use of major reference sources, in-house catalogs, CD-ROM resources, MEDLINE, and other electronic bibliographic indexes is also necessary to verify incomplete or incorrect citations and can be accomplished by using manuals or attending local training classes. ILL staff should also be adept in the using Locator for verifying bibliographic information and obtaining unique identification (UI) numbers for books, serials, and journal articles which are used to expedite the transmission of borrowing requests on DOCLINE. The bibliographic verification skills acquired for ILL are also useful at the reference desk, and highly knowledgeable and skilled ILL support staff will also assist there when needed. Interlibrary loan is a subject often included in workshop programs and classes sponsored by local, state, and regional groups, Regional Medical

Libraries, and other agencies to provide basic orientation and training for health sciences library staff.

Interlibrary Loan Policies

A comprehensive statement of interlibrary loan policy should exist in all health sciences libraries. Such a statement differs for each institution and reflects the particular needs, goals, and reciprocal commitments of the library. The interlibrary loan policy of a health sciences library should clearly designate the scope and goals of service, as well as people, agencies, and networks to be served and the library's responsibilities as a borrower and a lender. Policies should explain how services are to be funded and charged, detail relevant provisions of the copyright law, and describe the relationships of interlibrary loan functions to other library services and programs. These determinations are critical policy decisions that all health sciences libraries must make, and as such should be approved and reviewed regularly by appropriate administrative authorities within the library or parent institution. ILL policies should be documented and available to the library staff, appropriate lending libraries, and to library users.

Borrowing Policies

Because of differing requirements and responsibilities of the borrowing and lending functions, it is useful to develop separate policy statements for each. Borrowing policies should delineate who is eligible to use interlibrary loan (most libraries limit ILL borrowing to primary users); should indicate when it is appropriate to borrow materials (including whether or not materials in circulation, at the bindery, or missing are requested); and should specify the types of materials (e.g., rare manuscripts, bulky or fragile items, or material with local circulation restrictions) that can or cannot be requested. In addition, borrowing policies should state what protocols and transmission routes the library normally uses to obtain materials and point out any charges that may be incurred as a result of lending library fees.

Lending Policies

Lending policies should specify eligible libraries and the services to which they are entitled and indicate loan periods, routine and expedited charges, renewal protocol, and the method for delivery and return of ILL materials. Policies should also detail the types and formats of materials that circulate through ILL. If possible, lending policies should be placed in printed and online directories and sent to libraries that borrow materials frequently.

Special formats, such as media, machine-readable data files, and rare and unique materials, require special guidelines for shared access. Factors governing the loan of special formats include cost of the material, availability of replacement, condition of the original, impact on the lending library's primary user, and copyright and licensing restrictions. Special formats also have special access requirements such as on-site use in the borrowing library only or use in a classroom or campus media center. The borrowing library is responsible for adhering to any copyright and licensing regulations or other conditions which may apply to the use of loaned materials and for ensuring the safe return of materials to the lender.

The library's interlibrary lending policies should complement its circulation policies. In practice, health sciences libraries typically lend monographs, limit the circulation of serials, fill journal article requests with photocopies, and restrict renewals for materials circulated on ILL. Lending policies should strive to balance the needs of primary users with a commitment to resource sharing. Participating as a lending library should not substantially reduce the services rendered to primary users, even though a high-volume ILL service will inevitably remove a significant number of items from the shelf as well as increase reshelving work and collection wear and tear. If primary users are suffering from competition with interlibrary loan users for use of library materials, then the needs of the library's primary user should be given priority over the needs of the ILL user. It is important to remember, however, that resource sharing depends upon a willingness to reciprocate. Primary users will increasingly need to access and use external collections, and their ability to do so will be potentially diminished if more and more network participants develop overly restrictive ILL policies.

Lending policies should also specify charges for routine and expedited requests and provide guidelines for collecting fees. Policies should also describe billing procedures, payment requirements, and options such as departmental recharge accounts, deposit accounts, purchased coupons, credit cards, and contracts.

Policies and practices governing the use of telefacsimile transmission of items requested via ILL also need to be enumerated, as the use of this technology is definitely an emerging option for health sciences libraries and because its use has increased the workloads of ILL units [65]. Telefacsimile policies are still in the developmental phase, and if such policies exist at all, they vary greatly in terms of fees, circumstances under which libraries will initiate transmissions, and handling practices. Some libraries use fax transmission only for patient care emergencies, while others consider its use standard operating procedure. A number of libraries consider all fax borrowing requests to be rush requests and therefore process and bill accordingly; others distinguish between rush fax requests and simple fax requests and handle the latter as part of normal work flow. Fax borrowing requests via DOCLINE are usually processed by the lending library as part of the normal workload unless the request is actually marked rush.

Almost all lending libraries charge a surcharge for fax transmission to offset increased telecommunications costs and additional labor costs. Because of the cost implications to the user, the fax policies and fee schedules of lending libraries should be consulted prior to requesting a fax transmission.

Policies of Other Libraries, Networks, and the NN/LM

It is important to know what the lending policies of other libraries are, and this information can be obtained by periodically collecting individual policy statements from frequently used libraries or by consulting online ILL policy directories, such as DOCUSER and the OCLC Name-Address Directory, or the *Interlibrary Loan Policies Directory* [66]. Borrowing and lending responsibilities that apply to requests between libraries with no specific agreements are fully described in the "National Interlibrary Loan Code for the United States, 1993" [67] and the *Interlibrary Loan Practices Handbook* [68]. It is also important to obtain and update pertinent loan codes of local, system, and regional networks to which the library belongs. Because most health sciences libraries participate in the NN/LM, the policies of both the Resource and Regional Medical Libraries and the NLM should also be readily available. A regional ILL/document delivery policy manual is generally available through the various Regional Medical Libraries upon request.

The ILL policies, procedures, and practices of the NN/LM greatly affect all health sciences libraries because they establish criteria for requester eligibility, routing protocol, online network participation, ILL charges, cost containment, and performance standards. Each Regional Medical Library is responsible for developing and implementing a regional interlibrary loan policy, maintaining regional locator data and tools, coordinating access services to unaffiliated health professionals, and monitoring ILL performance data for the region. In accordance with the practices and requirements of NN/LM, health sciences libraries refer routine ILL requests to libraries close geographically to the borrowing library, a practice which reduces costs, expedites requests, and keeps larger net-lender libraries from being inundated with requests. Routine requests are then filled along hierarchial lending lines. If requests cannot be filled at the local level, they can be referred first to the Resource Library and then to the Regional Medical Library. If requested journals and books are not available in a designated region, they can be requested directly from the National Library of Medicine. Participation in the NN/LM also requires involvement in a number of related activities, such as contributing to union lists or databanks and the periodic compilation of statistical reports and analyses that are useful to network operations.

Performance Measures for Access Services

More and more libraries are beginning to analyze their activities quantitatively to better understand, manage, and improve operations and services. The use of performance measures to gather and analyze objective data is valuable to both large and small health sciences libraries. Measurement tools are useful in planning, decision making, problem solving, improving efficiency, demonstrating performance levels and resource needs, and in measuring the impact and effectiveness of library activities.

A wide variety of measurement tools such as input, process, productivity, output, and outcome have been used in libraries [69]. Although most performance measures have been developed and used in large academic libraries, many of them can be adapted to smaller libraries, including hospital libraries. Small service units or libraries, however, must be cautioned that extremely small samples or occasional activity may affect the validity of the results.

In choosing which tools to use, it is important to select those measures that most appropriately meet the specific needs of the library, unit, or service. Important questions to ask are why is the information needed and which data will be the most useful for the decision or problem at hand. Once performance measures are selected, used, and analyzed, it is beneficial to replicate the data collection process periodically in order to track any changes and determine improvement or decline.

The use of performance measures is very helpful in evaluating the extensiveness and effectiveness of access services delivered to users. Whitlach notes that numerous access studies have been conducted over the past twenty years using a variety of output measurements [70]. These addressed a wide variety of issues including accessibility and use of information resources, physical access to libraries, and physical retrieval of material from libraries, among other aspects. Some of the more important research studies confirm the importance of accessibility in information source use and selection [71]. Others have determined performance rates for institutions regarding document availability and have analyzed the major barriers to document availability such as circulation status, stacks maintenance error, and user bookstacks error [72]. One such book availability study showed that the performance scores of health sciences libraries were similar to those of general academic libraries [73]. Another important study discussed earlier compared the impact of uniform and variable loan periods on book use and selection [74].

The primary purpose of evaluating interlibrary loan service through the use of performance measures is to determine if services benefit library users. This determination can be made by using a variety of output measures, such as turnaround time and fill rate, to establish the quality and effectiveness of service. It is important to examine the ILL service from the user's perspective, and measures should be developed that address services delivered to users rather than to intermediate processes within the library required to deliver those services. For example, the measurement of turnaround time should measure the time from the material's initial request date to the date it was available to the borrower, not to the date the material arrived in the library for further processing; also, time measured should correspond to calendar days rather than the working days of ILL staff. Using measurement tools to quantify increases in workload and justify additional resources for ILL, another commonly used application, was discussed earlier under ILL staffing.

Because of the emphasis on speed and success in medical resource sharing, and because the use of ILL materials may be critical in patient care settings, interlibrary lending in health sciences libraries is one of the few areas of library service where performance standards have been rather widely introduced. The NN/LM, specifically the Regional Medical Libraries, regularly reviews the performance data provided by DOCLINE and other separate reports to determine acceptable minimum levels of performance for Resource and Regional Medical Libraries. These libraries must maintain a fulfillment (fill rate) standard of 75% and a throughput (turnaround time) standard which requires the processing of 85% of filled loans within four calendar days and the processing of 85% of nonavailable requests within seven calendar days.

Another common type of output measure concerns the satisfaction of key library constituencies and assesses the degree to which user needs are met. Performance assessment measures of this type employ user reports or surveys. Numerous approaches and measurement instruments have been developed that evaluate both the full scope of library activities and specific library services. Many studies incorporate methodologies for evaluating information access and availability and include indicators for materials availability, interlibrary loan, and the provision of equipment and facilities [75]. Considerations for developing user surveys include identifying performance criteria, adapting sample surveys from other libraries, developing a survey instrument that contains concise and relevant questions that evoke unbiased responses and that provides clear instructions, establishing a time frame and administration protocols, and compiling and analyzing the data. Both academic and hospital libraries are increasingly using surveys and needs assessment tools to improve quality continuously and to meet accreditation requirements. Both the *1995 Accreditation Manual For Hospitals* [76] and the MLA *Standards for Hospital Libraries* [77] require that hospital libraries regularly assess the information needs of the institution to measure and monitor library performance.

Recent changes in the economic environment and heightened concerns with institutional accountability in all library sectors have motivated a number of libraries to assess the productivity of internal library operations. These studies, in contrast to evaluative or performance measures, attempt to relate staff performance to expenditures or the number of staff to measures of service. The acute emphasis on accountability and productivity in hospitals prompted Phillips to develop productivity measures for a hospital library in an effort to demonstrate the need for, and value of, hospital library services in quantitative terms meaningful to administrators [78]. Phillips recommended that more studies of this nature be undertaken for gaining administrative visibility and support despite the high risks and suggested the need for balancing productivity studies with qualitative evaluations so as not to contain costs at the expense of quality service [79].

In developing reliable, valid, and precise measures for various health sciences library services, several excellent works are available that provide practical assistance in conducting meaningful measurements with minimum expense and difficulty. ALA's manual, *Measuring Academic Library Performance* [80], is instructional in nature and provides actual forms which have been tested and detailed directions for using output measures to evaluate major library services such as access and information services and facilities. Doelling's description of a model for planning and executing a user survey in an academic health sciences library, which includes a basic survey instrument, is also helpful [81]. Other excellent works focusing specifically on access services measurement and evaluation are Kantor's self-study manual [82] and the ARL Office of Management Services study of interlibrary loan workload and staffing [83].

It is important that health sciences librarians develop a knowledge base of performance measures and information services research for a variety of reasons. Increasingly, librarians are called upon to locate and evaluate research-based information from the literature to assist clinical decision making. It is also widely recognized that librarians need to increase their own research activity to establish effective, research-based information practices and services and to enhance their stature and influence as a profession. Recent developments of JCAHO and the education and research policies of the Medical Library Association underscore the importance of using research data in designing, managing, and improving patient, organizational, and library processes. Because evidence-based information is becoming central to both health care and the profession, it is now essential that health sciences librarians acquire skills to assume expanded research roles.

Copyright Implications of Access Services

As libraries move from collection building toward information access, library ownership of materials will decrease and the need to access the resources of others through library resource sharing and alternative electronic sources will increase. Moreover, declining budgets will force libraries to subsidize operations, services, and collections through cost recovery efforts. A library's ability to provide information access and fulfill its mission, however, may be significantly affected by legal considerations surrounding information access and copyrighted works. In the future, one of the biggest challenges confronting libraries will be how the evolving copyright law impacts access and use of library collections, especially electronic formats, and how it will apply to libraries' resource sharing and cost recovery efforts.

The following review of copyright issues provides background on the federal copyright law adopted by Congress in 1976, its subsequent amendments, and related guidelines. It discusses the copyright implications of various library services and activities, including interlibrary loan, photocopy and fee-based services, reserves, and access to media and computer files. Recent copyright developments and future professional actions are also described.

Copyright Act of 1976 and CONTU Guidelines

The United States copyright statute, fully revised in 1976, updated the outmoded copyright law of 1909. The Copyright Act of 1976 was designed to bring the law up to date and to consolidate and clarify existing law in light of new media and new transfer technologies [84]. This copyright law gives copyright owners exclusive rights to publish and use their original works (Section 106). Such exclusive rights, however, can limit the use of works by others, including librarians needing to duplicate materials for users and preservation, for faculty members requiring copied articles for classroom distribution, and for researchers and students using photocopies for personal study. Consequently the revised statute allows for the "fair use" of copyrighted works primarily for research and educational purposes, setting forth criteria to be considered in determining whether a given use is a "fair use" that will shield the user from copyright infringement liability (Section 107). The criteria include 1) the purpose and character of the use, 2) the nature of the work, 3) the amount or portion of material being used, and 4) the effect of the use upon the potential market. In addition, this law grants certain rights of reproduction specific to libraries and archives that are not covered under "fair use" (Section 108). Section 108 initially required that every five years the Copyright Office sponsor reviews or reports to Congress on the effects of the Section 108 provision; Congress subsequently received reports in 1983 and 1988, and in 1992 it repealed the requirement of further studies. This important law, which seeks to balance the interests of authors, publishers, and the public, has given rise to tremendous complexity and interpretation.

The 1976 copyright law is best understood when used in conjunction with several federal documents and guidelines. While these materials do not carry the force of law, they are considered in judicial interpretation, and they also assist librarians, educators, and others to better apply the law. Of particular note is the work of the Commission on New Technological Uses of Copyrighted Works (CONTU), which was set up to study copyright issues in light of new technologies and to recommend relevant changes to the copyright law. The "CONTU Guidelines on Photocopying and Interlibrary Arrangements" emerged as one the commission's most lasting achievements and still provide guidance to librarians and educators in understanding permissible limits of photocopying in the most commonly encountered library photocopying situations [85]. The commission also recommended to Congress relevant changes to the 1976 law regarding computer technology and, based on the commission's final recommendations, Congress amended the law in 1980. The resulting Computer Software Copyright Act of 1980 [86] defined "computer programs" and made the 1976 act applicable to computer programs as well. All of these documents and developments help explain various provisions of the copyright act which govern the rights and privileges of authors, publishers, instructors, scholars, researchers, and librarians.

A detailed statement of recommended practices to ensure compliance with the law and still maintain good service is presented in *The Copyright Law and the Health Sciences Librarian* [87]. This MLA publication includes pertinent sections of the law and related guidelines and federal regulations. The Gasaway guide is also comprehensive and informative [88]. In addition, the U.S. Copyright Office [89] and the American Library Association [90-94] have prepared publications that provide valuable assistance in explaining the provisions of the law and guidelines. Copyright-related works should be available in all health sciences libraries and consulted when questions arise.

Copyright and ILL

Copyright law has a direct bearing on interlibrary loan services and establishes different requirements for borrowing and lending libraries. Because most libraries perform both borrowing and lending functions, depending on circumstance, it is important that ILL staff be apprised of all pertinent copyright obligations. The copyright responsibilities of the borrowing library exceed those of the lending library because the law makes the borrowing library responsible for certain aspects of copyright compliance. Borrowing requirements discussed in the copyright act and related CONTU guidelines include copyright warning notification, systematic reproduction, copyright representation for requests, and record maintenance for interlibrary borrowing requests.

Section 108 of the copyright law requires a library to post a Display Warning of Copyright at all locations where borrowing requests are accepted and to include the same warning, an Order Warning of Copyright, on all borrowing request forms. The text of both notices is prescribed by regulation of the Register of Copyrights and must read [95]:

NOTICE
WARNING CONCERNING COPYRIGHT RESTRICTIONS

The copyright law of the United States (Title 17, United States Code) governs the making of photocopies or other reproductions of copyrighted material.

Under certain conditions specified in the law, libraries and archives are authorized to furnish a photocopy or other reproduction. One of these specified conditions is that the photocopy or reproduction is not to be "used for any purpose other than private study, scholarship, or research." If a user makes a request for, or later uses, a photocopy or reproduction for purposes in excess of "fair use," that user may be liable for copyright infringement.

This institution reserves the right to refuse to accept a copying order if, in its judgment, fulfillment of the order would involve violation of the copyright law.

The regulation states that the Display Warning sign should be printed on durable paper, be at least eighteen points in size, and be displayed prominently within the immediate vicinity where ILL orders are accepted.

The Order Warning notice on the printed ILL form should be noticeably printed within a box with type no smaller than eight points [96].

Since the copyright law was passed in 1976, many libraries no longer require users to come to the library to place interlibrary loan requests. Today users are frequently given options of requesting materials by voice mail, electronic mail, or telefacsimile transmission. Gasaway cautions that, in these cases, librarians need to find new creative ways to display this warning and comply with Section 108 notice stipulations. She suggests a number of possible approaches, such as verbally reading the warning over the telephone, telefaxing the warning to users, and programming a warning screen into e-mail and ILL systems, that should excuse the library from liability [97].

Section 108 also recognizes a library's right to participate in interlibrary arrangements so long as the "aggregate quantities" of articles borrowed through ILL do not substitute for a subscription or purchase of the work. The specific definition of "aggregate quantities" is addressed in the CONTU guidelines, with respect to the proviso at Section 108 (g)(2), which limits reproduction of copyright material that may be requested without special arrangements with copyright owners. These CONTU guidelines apply to periodical titles, not individual issues, cover only titles published within five years from the date of the ILL request, and permit the borrowing library to receive five articles per year from a title. Articles more than five years old from the time of the request are not subject to the guidelines' restrictions. These interlibrary borrowing provisions of the CONTU guidelines are commonly referred to as the "rule of five," although Gasaway has argued for the use of the phrase, "suggestion of five," to better distinguish them from federal law [98]. The provision for materials other than periodicals is similar except that the copying restriction is not for the prior five years but the entire period for which the work is copyrighted.

The borrowing library can also order copies of articles if it has ordered the title for purchase or if it owns the title, but the issue is not on the shelf, is missing, or is at the bindery when the user needs an article from it. Such requests are permissible exceptions to the "suggestion of five" under the CONTU guidelines.

Borrowing libraries are responsible for making sure that requests comply with the copyright law or the CONTU guidelines. To assure the lending library that the requests conform, the borrowing library must note compliance on the interlibrary loan request form and include the corresponding codes, either CCG (Conforms to Copyright Guidelines) or CCL (Conforms to Copyright Law). Unless these codes are included, the lending library must return the request unprocessed.

Because of record keeping requirements set forth in the guidelines, borrowing libraries must also maintain borrowing records for a certain period of time. Records for filled ILL photocopy requests that fall under the CONTU guidelines must be maintained for the current year plus the three previous calendar years. Libraries should also routinely discard older ILL records to avoid maintenance of excessive files and to help protect user confidentiality. Because the guidelines require that the number of photocopied items from a given journal or book received in the current year be known before another request for the same title is sent, it is necessary to keep a file or log arranged alphabetically by title and within title by year of publication. It is also important to remember that some publications are exempt from copyright protection, such as public domain materials and certain research reports funded by some federal agencies. Such publications, which usually include statements to this effect in the preliminary pages of the journal or article, may be copied without inclusion in the "suggestion of five." This information also appears in the MEDLINE record as the check tags SUPPORT, U.S. GOV'T, P.H.S. and SUPPORT, U.S. GOV'T, NON-P.H.S.

Libraries presented with ILL requests apparently in violation of the CONTU guidelines might wish to find appropriate alternatives for users to obtain the needed materials, even though these may lie outside customary interlibrary services. Some of the options available to ILL borrowers when they are about to or have exceeded the limit of five include borrowing an entire volume or issue from a willing lender; writing directly to the copyright holder for permission to copy or for reprints; placing a subscription to the journal if appropriate; referring the user to other local libraries that hold the title; purchasing the issue from the publisher or company which deals with back issues; purchasing a copy from a commercial document supplier that pays royalties on each journal article supplied; or if a library uses the Transactional Reporting Service of the Copyright Clearance Center (CCC) it can initiate an ILL request to other libraries and pay royalty fees to the CCC. In choosing the most appropriate course of action, each option should be weighed against the cost of use and the delays in service that may occur. Copyright considerations need not deny anyone access to information, but occasionally requesters and librarians may have to turn to nonlibrary sources for purchase of material or to make a royalty payment. Given shrinking book budgets, canceled periodical subscriptions, and the continuing growth in the number of periodicals published, it is likely that borrowing libraries will be asked more and more to provide alternative means of obtaining materials which exceed the "suggestion of five" limitations.

The lending library also has certain obligations under the copyright law and CONTU guidelines. Lending libraries are responsible for filling only requests that bear a copyright compliance declaration (CCL/CCG) from the requesting library. They are also responsible for maintaining reasonable supervision of interlibrary photocopying and for refraining from filling requests that appear to violate the law or the guidelines. In addition, each photocopy made at the lending library must include in a prominent place a notice that the material may be protected by copyright law. The American Library Association has recommended the following language [99]:

NOTICE
This material may be protected by
copyright law (Title 17, U.S. Code)

With the increase in telefacsimile transmission of ILL documents between libraries, a question arises concerning the use of a photocopy to transmit an article. In most ILL telefacsimile situations, the lender photocopies the material to be transmitted and temporarily retains the original photocopy while the borrower receives a copy via fax. The specific copyright issue in this practice concerns whether or not the original photocopy, which stays with the lender, constitutes a violation of the copyright law and CONTU guidelines, as the guidelines specifically state that a library may reproduce and distribute only a single copy of copyrighted material. Recent discussion of the issue in the library literature equates the production of a copy for fax transmission to the maintenance of a computer program second copy which is allowed under the copyright law [100-101]. Ensign concludes that by inference the original photocopy is not an infringement so long as it is not used for another purpose [102]. It is also recommended that the photocopy be destroyed after transmission to lessen telefax-related liability.

The same principle also applies when a lending library electronically scans an ILL document for network transmission to a borrowing library as with the Ariel document transmission system. As long as the scanned document is deleted from electronic storage after a successful transmission has occurred, the lender most likely is not in violation of copyright law, because the borrowing library received a single copy of copyrighted material, albeit an electronic copy. Gasaway points out that the electronic nature of library copying does not alter its copyright or fair use status [103]. To help avoid copyright liability in connection with new transfer technologies, libraries should develop written policy statements for telefacsimile, scanning, and network transmission procedures in consultation with legal counsel and include them in ILL policies.

Copyright and Photocopy Services

If libraries maintain self-service photocopy equipment on the premises for library users or for staff use, a warning notice must be placed on or near the equipment as required by Section 108 (f)(1) of the copyright law. Recommended wording for the notice is [104]:

NOTICE
WARNING CONCERNING COPYRIGHT RESTRICTIONS

The copyright law of the United States (Title 17, United States Code) governs the making of photocopies and other reproductions of copyrighted material. The person using this equipment is liable for any infringement.

This notice protects the library from liability for copyright infringement that may result from the unsupervised use of photocopy equipment in the library.

In situations where the library staff produces photocopies of library materials for users, as in the case of many hospital libraries, Section 108 requires that a warning of copyright as prescribed by the Register of Copyrights be displayed on the order forms and also posted on or near the equipment. If the ordering of photocopies is done electronically by users, the messaging system should include a copyright warning notification screen. The language of the warning notice is the same as that for the ILL notice described in the previous section. Mediated photocopy services should follow the "one article" rule which permits the library to make a single copy of an article or a small part of a copyrighted work. These copies must then become the property of the user. Libraries are sometimes permitted to photocopy from their collections entire works or substantial parts of works for primary users, if a copy cannot be obtained at a fair price. Multiple copy reproduction for reserve collections or classroom use is discussed in the section on copyright and reserves.

Copyright and Fee-Based Document Delivery

Fee-based document delivery services in academic libraries include a wide range of activities that encompass traditional interlibrary loan and in-house mediated photocopying services, specialized distribution services to primary users, and document delivery services to off-campus users. To offset the increasing costs of providing these services, academic libraries have traditionally charged both their primary and secondary users. Recently, however, some university libraries have established separate large-scale, well-publicized fee-based service units to handle requests from primarily off-campus users.

The copyright implications of these newly emerging fee-based document delivery services are uncertain, confusing, and controversial. Legal opinion differs as to what photocopy permissions are granted to libraries under these circumstances. In addition, practice differs as to how copyright compliance is achieved among university libraries with fee-based document delivery units. Because issues related to fee-based services are complex and because legal opinion and library practice vary, fee-based document delivery service policies and practices should be reviewed by legal counsel before initiating services.

In establishing policies and practices for these services and determining whether copying is permitted without first having to request permission or pay royalties, libraries need to consider several issues. Heller suggests that the entire operation be reviewed in order to determine whether this type of use is fair under the Section 107 criteria and whether these services would qualify for an exemption or in fact constitute an infringement according to "multiple or systematic copying" prohibitions in Section 108 [105]. Heller recommends that the library evaluate such factors as quantity of copying performed, extent of advertising activity, and revenue uses among other aspects [106]. Bunting contends that in-house document delivery services using resources from the library's own collection fall within fair use [107]. This interpretation is based on the fact that most, if not all, fee-based service operations are not making a profit but merely recovering partial costs. Therefore, these services qualify for the Section 108 exemption in that there is no "commercial advantage" in maintaining these services. This view has been challenged by the publishing community in an Association of American Publishers circular that considers library sponsored fee-based services to be indistinguishable from commercial suppliers [108].

More troublesome in terms of copyright is the practice of securing external resources from other libraries for community users. Bunting maintains that the provisions of Section 108 do not apply to this practice and that the obtaining of information for external users from outside sources may likely be deemed an infringement [109]. The practice also raises the issue of external community users possibly depriving the library's primary clientele of needed interlibrary loan materials by exhausting CONTU "suggestion of five" limitations.

Libraries handle copyright issues related to document delivery services differently depending on differing operations, environments, and interpretations of the law. Health sciences libraries in for-profit environments, such as pharmaceutical companies and for-profit hospitals, may be required either to obtain permissions from copyright owners or use the convenient option of seeking a blanket authorization license from the CCC, even when copying materials from their own collections. Some educational institutions do so to reduce possible liability for copyright infringement. Other educational institutions view the copying of their collections as allowable and do not obtain permissions or pay royalty fees. Most academic libraries make royalty payments to the CCC on a per transaction basis or use commercial document suppliers when obtaining materials from external sources for secondary users. For additional information on the legal considerations of fee-based document delivery services in health sciences libraries, librarians should consult Bunting's article [110].

Copyright and Reserves

The 1976 copyright legislation bears directly upon the reserve room practices of many libraries, as reserve collections traditionally provide multiple copies of materials (articles or portions of monographs) to students as part of their required classwork. Section 107 specifically states that reproduction of a copyrighted work for teaching, including multiple copies for classroom use, is not an infringement of copyright if the use of the materials complies with the fair use criteria set forth in the law. In addition, multiple copying for classroom use is addressed in the related guidelines, "Agreement on Guidelines for Classroom Copying in Not-For-Profit Educational Institutions with Respect to Books and Periodicals," which were drawn up by a group of affected parties to define further fair use in classroom situations [111]. The guidelines state that this type of copying must meet the tests of "brevity," "spontaneity," and "cumulative effect" and that each copy include a notice of copyright.

Multiple copy reproduction of copyrighted materials in reserve collections is customarily handled by either the library or the faculty member. If the library performs the photocopying, copying should be done in accordance with fair use guidelines governing classroom use. If this is not the case, libraries should seek permission from copyright owners to make multiple copies of materials or make appropriate payments to the Academic Permissions Service of the CCC for the multiple copies made. Faculty members may request that their personal collections of single or multiple photocopies be placed on reserve for students. If this happens, the library should insist that the copies be labeled as the personal property of the individual faculty member. Some libraries even require the faculty member to sign a form indicating that he or she provided the copies. Faculty copies placed on reserve also have to meet the requirements of the copyright law; however, the burden of adherence to copyright is placed on the faculty member rather than the library. Some libraries are beginning to scan reserve documents into machine readable form and to make them accessible through circulating disks or networks. While "fair use" described in the guidelines applies to reserve copying irrespective of format, the library should carefully weigh the copyright implications before implementing electronic reserves projects and should move toward an electronic environment following the guidelines as closely as possible. For additional information regarding copyright and reserves, librarians should consult *The Copyright Law and the Health Sciences Librarian* [112].

Copyright and Audiovisuals

As with printed library materials, it is important to be aware of the legal guidelines that apply to the use of audiovisual materials in libraries, specifically to the in-house use, the lending, and the copying of audiovisuals in a library collection. When establishing appropriate policies and practices for audiovisuals, librarians need to use good judgment and apply fair use principles as delineated in the copyright law. Librarians should also review the advisory statements of various library associations and other authoritative sources regarding the use of audiovisuals in libraries and obtain legal counsel when necessary [113-118].

Of particular interest to health sciences libraries is the use and copying of purchased videotapes in libraries because these have become a common part of the collections of both academic and hospital libraries. Proper legal practices regarding the in-house use of videotapes in libraries are somewhat uncertain because precise rules governing the showing or "public performance" of these materials in the library environment have yet to be established in a court of law. Despite this ambiguity, it is generally believed that individual viewing of videotapes on library-owned equipment within the library is permitted under the copyright law [119]. More problematic, however, is a group viewing situation in a library viewing room. It is probably acceptable for very small groups to view a videotape in a library study carrel or viewing room provided it is in the course of instruction [120-121]. Large group viewings, on the other hand, would need to comply with various educational stipulations set forth in Section 110. These conditions require, among other things, that the viewing take place in a classroom or similar place devoted to instruction of a nonprofit educational institution and that the viewing be connected with a face-to-face teaching activity.

If individual users view videotapes in a library, notices should be posted on the video playing equipment to educate and warn users that many videotapes are protected by copyright and that unauthorized copying is prohibited by law. Suggested American Library Association wording is [122]:

Many videotaped materials are protected by copyright. 17 U.S.C. Sec. 101. Unauthorized copying may be prohibited by law.

Videotapes, as well as other audiovisuals, in a library's collection may also be loaned to users for their personal use, but should not be knowingly loaned to groups for public performances. If audiovisuals are loaned to users for personal use, the copyright notice that appears on the work should not be obscured.

Under certain circumstances, libraries can also duplicate audiovisual materials for preservation and security purposes. Section 108 permits the reproduction of a published work for the purpose of replacing a damaged, deteriorated, lost, or stolen copy, if it cannot be obtained at a fair price after a reasonable effort. Some libraries consider reformatting and copying in anticipation of deterioration or damage to be acceptable library practice within copyright guidelines. Because the law pertaining to copying audiovisual material under these categories is complicated, libraries should seek a release from the owner of the copyright before proceeding to duplicate for these purposes. Instructors within nonprofit educational institutions may also record broadcast television programs for classroom use so long as they meet all of the retention and use standards set forth in the "Guidelines For Off-Air Recording Of Broadcast Programming Works For Educational Purposes" [123].

Much of what has been described above concerns the fair use of audiovisuals purchased for a library collection. Libraries also need to be aware of contractual conditions frequently attached to new audiovisual purchases, since many such conditions purport to prohibit the exercise of fair use rights under Section 107. Often the conditions will grant the purchaser fewer rights than are accorded under copyright law and may necessitate the specialized handling of each audiovisual if the terms of a given license are accepted by the library. Van Vuren and Kwak urge librarians to review carefully the licensing terms of audiovisuals as these may affect internal library operations and limit user access to these materials [124]. Librarians will need to contact producers and distributors if provisions fail to meet user needs as is frequently the case. If necessary, letters to producers of audiovisuals should request duplication rights for archival purposes, conversion rights so that material can be periodically updated to standard formats, and public performance rights within the library and on campus [125]. Another management practice that some libraries use when purchasing audiovisuals is to place conditions on their purchases of audiovisuals to help assure an agreement with the publisher about the work's intended use. This can be done by placing language on a purchase order that specifies how the library expects to use the work and that asserts the rights granted to libraries under Sections 107, 108, and 110 of the copyright law. Some examples of wording are available in the library literature and may be helpful for librarians to review prior to composing conditional purchasing statements for their libraries [126-127].

Copyright and Electronic Formats

Few specific legal guides exist to assist library managers in establishing access and use policies for machine-readable formats in library collections. Although the 1976 law was amended in 1980 to address computer programs, the amendment only minimally addressed computer issues and, to date, virtually no case law exists that clarifies computer usage in educational environments. More recently, however, Congress passed the Computer Software Rental Amendments Act of 1990 which exempts software from the "first sale" doctrine of the copyright law (Section 109) and makes it an infringement to rent, lease, or lend computer software for commercial purposes [128]. Notwithstanding the passage of this narrowly drafted act, the paucity of clear, specific legislation and legal precedents for software and database usage in education has created much uncertainty and misperception about what copyright restrictions and permissions may or may not apply.

In the absence of mandated legal practices, and until future statutes and legal precedents clarify rights, libraries should adopt informed, reasonable, and prudent policies and practices regarding software collections and database access. Management decisions should reflect the spirit of the copyright law in that policies should attempt to balance the rights of copyright owners and the needs of users and permit the fullest possible use of these materials under copyright law.

Responsible management practices in regards to the in-house use of software on library equipment involves allowing the use of a single program or copy of a program on one machine at a time. Libraries should purchase an original program for every circulating copy; each copy can be used repeatedly by different users on different machines as long as the usage is sequential and nonconcurrent. Single programs should not be loaded into a computer in such a way as to permit multiple simultaneous access of the program from several different terminals or computers. Mutually agreed upon license terms accompanying programs should be observed to avoid liability for breach of contract. Warning copyright notices should be posted on all unsupervised public-use microcomputers to avoid liability should users copy software illegally. Suggested American Library Association wording is [129]:

Many computer programs are protected by copyright, 17 U.S.C. 101. Unauthorized copying may be prohibited by law.

Some libraries take additional copyright notification measures and include electronic copyright warning messages on library software disks and on library networks. Other libraries have users sign statements indicating compliance with copyright laws as a condition for using library software and equipment. While these precautionary measures indicate a library's sensitivity in protecting the rights of the vendors, librarians should remember that the copyright law also protects libraries from inappropriate copying by users if copyright warning notices are appropriately displayed.

Because the Computer Software Rental Amendments Act exempts nonprofit libraries and educational institutions from lending restrictions, most health sciences libraries can circulate software outside the confines of the library. The act states that nonprofit libraries are allowed to lend software for nonprofit purposes, provided a copyright warning is affixed to the package of the circulating item. The text of this warning must read [130]:

NOTICE
WARNING OF COPYRIGHT RESTRICTIONS

The copyright law of the United States (Title 17, United States Code) governs the reproduction, distribution, adaptation, public performance, and public display of copyrighted material.

Under certain conditions of the law, nonprofit libraries are authorized to lend, lease, or rent copies of computer programs to patrons on a nonprofit basis and for nonprofit purposes. Any person who makes an unauthorized copy or adaptation of the computer program, or redistributes the loan copy, or publicly performs or displays the computer program, except as permitted by Title 17 of the United States Code, may be liable for copyright infringement.

This institution reserves the right to refuse to fulfill a loan request if, in its judgment, fulfillment of the request would lead to violation of the copyright law.

The Computer Software Rental Amendments Act contains a "sunset" provision and expires October 1, 1997. In March 1994, three years after the law's enactment, the Register of Copyrights submitted a report to Congress that evaluated the exemption and did not recommend any changes to the original act. Libraries should be aware that many software licensing conditions preclude the lending of software. In these cases the library should inform the vendor of the recent federal legislation and negotiate an improved agreement.

Section 117 stipulates that for collection maintenance purposes, libraries can lawfully make one archival copy provided that the copy is stored or archived, that only one copy is in use at any given time, and that the copy is destroyed if the library no longer owns the program. Archival copies should bear the appropriate copyright notices. Libraries can also make a copy of the original if the circulating copy is damaged, destroyed, or stolen.

Libraries should take a critical and proactive approach to licensing terms that accompany many software packages. The terms and conditions of the licenses frequently purport to extend protection provisions and exclude traditional fair use according to the federal copyright statutes. Many of these official-sounding licenses limit usage to one machine at a time, permit the making of a single backup, and prohibit lending; some may even require the signature of the librarian to verify that licensing conditions will be met. These licenses tend to favor software manufacturers, have questionable legal value, and contain provisions that are not in the best interests of library users [131-138].

For these reasons librarians should thoroughly examine each software license. If a license is overly restrictive, librarians should contact the producer and seek an agreement that meets the library and user needs at the time of purchase. McKirdy suggests that as a minimum requirement in library environments, software vendors should allow "multiple sequential users...to use the software nonconcurrently on different machines" [139]. Verbal understandings between the librarian and producer should be confirmed in writing soon after negotiations have concluded. Gasaway also suggests that a librarian can edit the text of a license by deleting detrimental clauses and inserting more favorable provisions and return it to the copyright holder [140]; the legal effect of such a practice will be based on the specific facts and circumstances involved. Some libraries place conditions on the purchases of software and routinely include statements on software purchase orders which specify library access practices and assert fair use rights granted to educational entities, such as libraries, under the copyright law [141]. On occasion librarians may need to negotiate formally contractual agreements where special fee schedules are established, such as site or network licenses. In these cases librarians should critically review the terms of the contract, assess each provision, and only sign if the agreement is reasonable, allows for sufficient access, and meets user needs. Valauskas cautions librarians to insist on reasonable use policies and not to compromise the "basic premises of fair use and the access rights of libraries" in an effort to secure expedient agreements [142].

Software licensing information, mutual agreements, contracts, and other pertinent information should be retained as part of the library's acquisition record. Acquisition records should indicate whether copyrighted or public domain software was purchased, whether multiple copies were obtained, whether licensing agreements were accepted or negotiated, and what terms and conditions were part of the agreement.

Recent Copyright Developments

Several recent court cases have generated significant discussion in the library literature. The first involves the 1991 Kinko's case [143] in which the court ruled that Kinko's Graphics Corporation had exceeded its rights of fair use when it photocopied textbook chapters for use at local universities. Of particular interest to the court was the profit motive of the Kinko's operation and the substantiality of the portions copied. While the Kinko's case raises some limited concerns about copyright on campus, i.e., the reliability of the "Classroom Guidelines" as a legally meaningful standard, this decision in no way overturns the fair use provisions of the 1976 law, particularly for nonprofit educational purposes.

Of more significance, however, is the 1992 Texaco decision that has the potential of setting legal precedent for fair use of copyrighted materials for research purposes in a corporate environment [144]. In this case the judge ruled that a Texaco scientist violated the copyright law's fair use provisions by copying single articles from various scientific journals to which the company subscribed. Similar to the Kinko's case, the most significant aspect in the court's determination was the underlying profit motive of the company. Despite Texaco's claim that such photocopying was a traditionally recognized example of fair use, the court held that the scientific research in question was commercial in nature since scientists were employed by a profit-seeking entity. The decision also dramatically elevated the role of the CCC in facilitating copyright permissions.

It has been suggested that the decision, if not overturned by a higher court, would significantly impact libraries in the for-profit sector because they would be subject to the findings of the case and prohibited from photocopying journal articles without obtaining permission or compensating the copyright holder [145]. Health sciences libraries most affected by the decision would be those of pharmaceutical companies and for-profit hospitals. While the Texaco case raises a number of issues about fair use in the for-profit sector, Crews maintains that a careful analysis of both decisions shows that the cases have limited application for nonprofit libraries and educational environments and cautions that libraries and universities should not misread the findings and make detrimental sacrifices of fair use privileges granted to most research libraries and universities [146].

The decision of the lower court in the Texaco case was appealed in May 1993. MLA, in coalition with six other organizations, filed an *amicus curiae* (friend of the court) brief in support of Texaco's appeal [147] because the ruling erodes the fair use privileges of all libraries and potentially impairs health information access and dissemination and thus patient care [148]. In October 1994, the second Circuit Court of Appeals upheld the decision of the lower court [149]. The appellate decision was based on somewhat different grounds than the original decision; the court affirmed the earlier decision because of the archival nature of the photocopying rather than the fact that Texaco was a for-profit company. In April 1995, shortly after the appellate ruling, Texaco petitioned the U.S. Supreme Court to review the important case. In May 1995, Texaco subsequently agreed to settle the lawsuit brought by the American Geophysical Union and several other publishers, thus eliminating the opportunity for the U.S. Supreme Court to review and possibly resolve the issues involved [150].

Librarians have been equally interested in a 1991 U.S. Supreme Court case involving copyright and compilations, a type of publication that includes most commercially significant databases and directories. The Court, in *Feist Publications, Inc. vs. Rural Telephone Service Co.,* ruled that a white pages listing of a telephone directory consisted of noncopyrightable facts arranged in an unoriginal manner and that copyright only protects works that are original [151]. The Court further noted that, in the case of compilations, originality exists in the "selection, coordination or arrangement" of the data and not in the data themselves. In addition, the court rejected the "sweat of the brow" analysis (the amount of effort undertaken to produce a work) as justification for copyright protection. In light of this decision, various attorneys, industry representatives, and librarians have predicted that information proprietors will increasingly use alternative legal measures, i.e., licenses and contracts, to ensure greater copyright protection [152-153]. In response to the important Supreme Court decision, the American Medical Association included a licensing agreement with the 33rd edition of the *Directory of Physicians in the United States.* This agreement restricted the use of the text to reference purposes, precluded its circulation outside the library and in library interlibrary programs, and prohibited photocopying of the directory. Due to the unprecedented and overly restrictive nature of the license, MLA on behalf of health sciences librarians and others negotiated an improved agreement with the American Medical Association in 1993. The new agreement limits librarians' responsibility for user copying in libraries if copyright warnings and notices are placed on library photocopy machines [154].

Future Directions

It is important, even imperative, for librarians to have a thorough understanding of the difficult legal issues surrounding copyrighted works, especially as they pertain to new technology. Knowledge of the basic provisions and purposes of copyright law is essential to apply copyright concepts to day-to-day library decisions and problems. Librarians also need to know about the privileges accorded libraries within the law and the rights of users of copyrighted materials so that they can challenge overly restrictive interpretations of the law, asserting fair use rights when necessary. Librarians will also need to propose reasonable and fair library and publishing practices and new copyright legislation with regards to emerging technologies.

Librarians can acquire this knowledge by reading the Copyright Act of 1976 and subsequent amendments, reviewing associated guidelines such as the CONTU guidelines, consulting MLA and ALA copyright advisory statements [155-157], and keeping current by reading copyright-related journal articles and books. An excellent legal treatise is *Nimmer on Copyright,* which is considered a leading authoritative reference work on copyright [158]. Librarians will also benefit greatly from reading *The Nature of Copyright: A Law of Users' Rights* [159], a primary copyright resource that examines the fair use doctrine and the balance of rights among authors, publishers, and users. In addition, libraries should seek the advice of qualified lawyers to establish a library's legal standing on any given matter.

Librarians must also educate the commercial owners of copyrights through direct license negotiations and by other means about the fair use rights of libraries. Certainly, librarians should resist entering into agreements that limit access rights to these materials granted to libraries under federal law. The publishing industry also needs to know of the commercial value of library collections as libraries are buyers and purveyors of their products. Matheson also points out that publishers and producers need to be aware of the preservation role of libraries and that libraries will be future sources of their out-of-print and obsolete products [160]. At the same time, librarians should demonstrate their sensitivity to the concerns of copyright holders by honoring the proprietary components of the copyright law and by disallowing violations no matter how widespread.

Libraries also need to take an assertive approach and develop strategies for ensuring that the "fragile fair use rights and privileges" of libraries are protected and to work towards their acceptance [161]. Crews suggests that libraries develop coordinated responses involving the entire professional and university communities [162]. He recommends that a widely accepted set of copyright standards for libraries be developed cooperatively, similar to the 1982 ALA photocopying model policy [163], and that libraries actively seek their endorsement by the U.S. Copyright Office and other diverse groups [164]. Other proposals that have been made seek to change established scholarly publishing practices which many believe favor the proprietary rights of publishers and producers. An informative overview of the various proposals appears in a journal article by Bennett [165]. Finally, librarians should be the "champions of the public interest" and use their knowledge and experience to take a leadership role in helping shape new copyright laws and regulations, so that legal access to copyrighted materials provides the flexibility and fairness that libraries and users require [166].

Conclusion

How access services as a concept and organizational model evolve in the future and whether the growing trend toward institutionalizing access services as a unit will be universally adopted in health sciences libraries is still a matter of question. That all health sciences libraries regardless of type, size, and resources will need to reexamine their goals and objectives in light of this dimension is not. Their vision of access services will probably parallel to a large extent developments that are underway in the academic and public library sectors, because health sciences libraries have been acutely interested in designing, delivering, and evaluating responsive and accessible information services for a long time.

It is most likely, however, that there will be significant differences in the medical model as a result of unique information issues. These issues include not only the need to incorporate quality practices in library management according to JCAHO requirements and health sciences library standards but also developments in medical informatics, evidence-based medicine and information, public policy regarding national health care, and the role of the National Information Infrastructure (NII) and NLM in the access and delivery of medical information sources and in supporting health sciences library operations. Moreover, the new marketplace of electronic information, with ever-increasing copyright restrictions and costs, is of particular concern to health sciences librarians, because restricted and unequal access to health information may impair medical education, research, and patient care, and thus the nation's health.

Sapp suggests that the vitality of the access concept rests in its versatility and its adaptability to differing realities and conditions [167]. It will be interesting to see how the model will be shaped by both hospital and academic health sciences library environments, whether it will provide an effective means of dealing with the opportunities and challenges that face the medical virtual library, and whether it will enhance access to and use of health literature by everyone.

References

1. Whitlatch JB. Access services. In: Lynch MJ, Young A, eds. Academic libraries: research perspectives. Chicago: American Library Association, 1990:67-105. (ACRL publications in librarianship no. 47).

2. Larsen PM. The climate of change: library organizational structures, 1985-1990. In: McCombs GM, ed. Access services: the convergence of reference and technical services. New York: Haworth Press, 1991:79-93. (The reference librarian no. 34).

3. Whitlatch, op. cit., 69.

4. Steel V. Access services: organization and management. Washington, DC: Association of Research Libraries, Office of Management Services, November/December 1991. (SPEC flyer 179).

5. Lessick SR. Access services. Message to: MEDLIB-L. In MEDLIB-L [Bitnet/Internet listserv] Start NE, list owner. Buffalo: State University of New York at Buffalo. 1992 Aug 13, 9:10 [28 lines].

6. Steel, op. cit.

7. Steel, op. cit.

8. Lange KS, Tietjen LD. Management challenges and issues in access services administration. In: Sapp G, ed. Access services in libraries: new solutions for collection management. New York: Haworth Press, 1992:37-61.

9. Lessick, op. cit.

10. Lessick, op. cit.

11. Carver D. From circulation to access services: the shift in academic library organization. In: Sapp G, ed. Access services in libraries: new solutions for collection management. New York: Haworth Press, 1992:23-36.

12. Ibid., 26-30.

13. Ibid., 30-34.

14. Jones CL, Kasses CD. Lending services: circulation policies, procedures, and problems. In: Darling L, Bishop D, Colaianni LA, eds. Handbook of medical library practice. 4th ed. v.1. Chicago: Medical Library Association, 1982:65-94.

15. Ibid., 91.

16. Young B. Circulation service: is it meeting the user's needs? J Acad Libr 1976 Jul;2(3):120-5.

17. Brian B. After hours access summary. Message to: MEDLIB-L. In MEDLIB-L [Bitnet/Internet listserv] Start NE, list owner. Buffalo: State University of New York at Buffalo. 1993 Jun 15, 14:57 [51 lines].

18. Paietta A, Fryer RK, Sette L. Access services staff: the solution for evening and weekend reference service. Med Ref Q 1993 Summer;12(2):35-43.

19. Young, op. cit., 121.

20. Bailey AS, Lennertz LL. The role of the access services manager in policy formation. In: Sapp G, ed. Access services in libraries: new solutions for collection management. New York: Haworth Press, 1992:119-32.

21. Ibid., 128-30.

22. Topper JM. Circulation and maintenance of library materials. In: Bradley J, Holst R, Messerle J, eds. Hospital library management. Chicago: Medical Library Association, 1983:88-101.

23. 1995 Accreditation manual for hospitals. Oakbrook Terrace, IL: Joint Commission on Accreditation of Healthcare Organizations, 1994:62.

24. Standards for hospital libraries. Chicago: Medical Library Association, 1994.

25. Hafner AW. A survey of patient access to hospital and medical school libraries. Bull Med Libr Assoc 1994 Jan;82(1):64-6.

26. Lyders RA. Task force drafts ethics code. MLA News 1994 Mar;(263):1,7.

27. Jones, op. cit., 75-6.

28. Buckland MK. An operations research study of a variable loan and duplication policy at the University of Lancaster. Libr Q 1972 Jan;42(1):97-106.

29. Annual statistics of medical school libraries in the United States & Canada, 1991-92. 15th ed. Houston: Association of Academic Health Sciences Library Directors, 1993:156-7.

30. Ibid., 156-7.

31. Lyders, op. cit., 7.

32. ALA Council adopts new code of ethics. Libr Pers News 1995 Sep/Oct;9(5):7.

33. Intellectual freedom manual. 4th ed. Chicago: American Library Association, 1992: 227-8.

34. Ibid., 228-9.

35. Ibid.

36. Lyons AG. Circulation policies, overdues, and fines: results of a survey of academic health sciences libraries. Bull Med Libr Assoc 1981 Jul;69(3):326-9.

37. DuBois HJ. From leniency to lockout: circulation policies at forty-three academic libraries. Coll Res Libr News 1986 Dec;47(11):698-702.

38. Hansel P, Burgin R. Hard facts about overdues. Libr J 1983 Feb 15;108(4):349-52.

39. Burgin R, Hansel P. More hard facts on overdues. Libr Arch Security 1984 Summer/Fall;6(2/3):5-17.

40. Burgin R, Hansel P. Library overdues: an update. Libr Arch Security 1990;10(2):51-75.

41. Little P. Managing overdues: facts from four studies. Bottom Line 1988;2(2):22-5.

42. Ibid., 23-5.

43. Burgin, Library overdues, op. cit., 74.

44. Ibid., 64.

45. Johnson CL. New realities in interlibrary cooperation: report on an ALA conference program. J Interlibr Loan Inf Supply 1991;2(1):73-6.

46. ARL statistics 1980-81: a compilation of statistics from the one hundred and thirteen members of the Association of Research Libraries. Washington, DC: Association of Research Libraries, 1981:18.

47. ARL statistics 1990-91: a compilation of statistics from the one hundred and nineteen members of the Association of Research Libraries. Washington, DC: Association of Research Libraries, 1992:31.

48. Annual statistics of medical school libraries in the United States & Canada, 1980-81. 4th ed. Houston: Association of Academic Health Sciences Library Directors, 1981:42.

49. Annual statistics of medical school libraries in the United States & Canada, 1990-91. 14th ed. Houston: Association of Academic Health Sciences Library Directors, 1992:88.

50. ARL statistics 1980-81, op. cit., 16.

51. ARL statistics 1990-91, op. cit., 29.

52. Lyon-Hartmann B. DOCLINE growth statistics: FY1985-FY1992 [informal compilation]. November 1992.

53. Rottmann FK. To buy or to borrow: studies of the impact of interlibrary loan on collection development in the academic library. J Interlibr Loan Inf Supply 1991;1(3):17-27.

54. Jackson ME. Library to library: fitting the bill. Wilson Libr Bull 1992 Jun;66(10):95-7.

55. Ibid., 95-7.

56. Ibid., 96.

57. Roche MM. ARL/RLG interlibrary loan cost study: a joint effort by the Association of Research Libraries and the Research Libraries Group. Washington, DC: Association of Research Libraries, 1993:iv.

58. Arcari RD. An overview of cost recovery. In: Wood MS, ed. Cost analysis, cost recovery, marketing, and fee-based services. New York: Haworth Press, 1985:71-81.

59. Ibid., 74-8.

60. Weaver-Meyers P, Clement S, Mahin C. Interlibrary loan in academic and research libraries: workload and staffing. Washington, DC: Association of Research Libraries, Office of Management Services, 1988:8. (Occasional paper OP15).

61. Ibid., 14.

62. Ibid., Appendix C.

63. National Library of Medicine. DOCLINE manual. Washington, DC: National Institutes of Health, 1989.

64. OCLC workbook: using the PRISM service. Dublin, OH: OCLC Online Computer Library Center, 1990.

65. Voyles JF, Cox JL. The impact of telefacsimile on interlibrary loan. J Interlibr Loan Inf Supply 1991;1(4):71-7.

66. Morris LR. Interlibrary loan policies directory. 5th ed. New York: Neal-Schuman, 1995.

67. National interlibrary loan code for the United States, 1993. RQ 1994 Summer;33(4):477-9.

68. Boucher V. Interlibrary loan practices handbook. 2nd ed. Chicago: American Library Association. In press.

69. Van House NA. Output measures in libraries. Libr Trends 1989 Fall;38(2):269-79.

70. Whitlatch, op. cit., 67-105.

71. Ibid., 70-1.

72. Manbridge J. Availability studies in libraries. Libr Inf Sci Res 1986 Oct/Dec;8(4):299-314.

73. Kolner SJ, Welch EC. The book availability study as an objective measure of performance in a health sciences library. Bull Med Libr Assoc 1985 Apr;73(2):121-131.

74. Buckland, op. cit., 97-106.

75. Van House, op. cit., 271-4.

76. 1995 Accreditation manual for hospitals, op. cit., 62.

77. Standards for hospital libraries, op. cit., 6-7.

78. Phillips SA. Productivity measurement in hospital libraries: a case report. Bull Med Libr Assoc 1990 Apr;78(2):146-153.

79. Ibid., 152-3.

80. Van House NA, Weil BT, McClure CR. Measuring academic library performance: a practical approach. Chicago: American Library Association, 1990.

81. Doelling DL. Blueprint for performance assessment. Med Ref Serv Q 1993 Spring;12(1):29-38.

82. Kantor PB. Objective performance measures for academic and research libraries. Washington, DC: Association of Research Libraries, 1984.

83. Weaver-Meyers, op. cit., 1-15, Appendix A-E.

84. Copyright act of 1976, Pub.L. No. 94-553, 90 Stat. 2541 (1976).

85. National Commission on New Technological Uses of Copyrighted Works. Guidelines for the proviso of subsection 108(g)(2), H.R. Rep. No. 1733, 94th Cong., 2d Sess. 69 (1976).

86. Computer software copyright act of 1980, Pub. L. No. 96-517, 94 Stat. 3015, 3028 (1980).

87. Copyright law and the health sciences librarian. Rev. ed. Chicago: Medical Library Association, 1989.

88. Gasaway LN, Wiant SK. Libraries and copyright: a guide to copyright law in the 1990s. Washington, DC: Special Libraries Association, 1994.

89. U.S. Library of Congress. Copyright Office. Publications on copyright. Washington, DC: Government Printing Office, April 1993. (Circular 2).

90. Reed MH. The copyright primer for librarians and educators. Chicago: American Library Association, 1987.

91. Model policy concerning college and university photocopying for classroom, research and library reserve use. Washington, DC: American Library Association, Washington Office, 1982.

92. Video and copyright. Chicago: American Library Association, 1992. (Library and information center fact sheet 7).

93. Telefacsimile and libraries: copyright issues. Chicago: American Library Association, 1991. (Library and information center fact sheet 16).

94. Computer software copyright warning. Chicago: American Library Association, 1993. (Library and information fact sheet 17).

95. 37 Code of federal regulations §201.14.

96. Ibid.

97. Gasaway LN. Copyright issues in electronic information and document delivery in special libraries. At Your Service 1993 Sep:10-13.

98. Gasaway LN. Copyright law in the age of technology [course sponsored by the University of Iowa]. Coralville, IA, September 13, 1993.

99. Warning notices for copies and machines. Am Libr 1977 Nov;8(10):530.

100. Schmidt SJ. The bogeyman: telefax and copyright. J Interlibr Loan Inf Supply 1991;2(1):5-7.

101. Ensign D. Copyright considerations for telefacsimile transmission of documents in interlibrary loan transactions. Law Libr J 1989 Fall;81(4):805-12.

102. Ibid., 811.

103. Gasaway, Copyright issues in electronic information, op. cit., 10.

104. Three words added to copyright notice. Am Libr 1978 Jan;9(1):22.

105. Heller JS. Copyright and fee-based copying services. Coll Res Libr 1986 Jan;47(1):28-37.

106. Ibid., 33.

107. Bunting A. Legal considerations for document delivery services. Bull Med Libr Assoc 1994 Apr;82(2):183-7.

108. Association of American Publishers. Statement of the Association of American Publishers on commercial and fee-based document delivery. New York: The Association, 1992.

109. Bunting, op. cit., 184.

110. Bunting, op. cit.

111. Agreement on guidelines for classroom copying in not-for-profit educational institutions with respect to books and periodicals, H.R. Conf. Rep. No. 1476, 94th Cong., 2d Sess. 68 (1976).

112. Copyright law and the health sciences librarian, op. cit., 7.

113. Ibid., 2-3.

114. Reed, op. cit., 29-43.

115. Video and copyright, op. cit.

116. Hemnes TM, Pyle AH. A guide to copyright issues in higher education. Washington, DC: National Association of College and University Attorneys, 1991.

117. Bielefield AC, Cheeseman LG. Libraries and copyright law. New York: Neal-Schuman, 1993. (Libraries and the law series).

118. Scholtz JC. Video policies and procedures for libraries. Santa Barbara, CA: ABC-CLIO, 1991.

119. Video and copyright, op. cit.

120. Ibid.

121. Hemnes, op. cit., 12.

122. Video and copyright, op. cit.

123. 127 Cong. Rec. 24049 (daily ed. April 14, 1981).

124. Van Vuren DD, Kwak AR. Audiovisual licensing: purchasing is not owning. J Biocomm 1986 Winter;13(1):22-5.

125. Gasaway, Copyright law in the age of technology, op. cit.

126. Copyright law and the health sciences librarian, op. cit., 3.

127. Scholtz, op. cit., 156.

128. Computer software rental amendments act of 1990. Pub. L. No. 101-650, §801, 104 Stat. 5134-5137 (1990).

129. Reed MH, Stanek D. Library and classroom use of copyrighted videotapes and computer software. Am Libr 1986 Feb;17(2):4p insert between 120-1.

130. Computer software copyright warning, op. cit.

131. Demas S. Copyright and legal considerations. In: Curtis C, ed. Public access microcomputers in academic libraries: the Mann Library model at Cornell University. Chicago: American Library Association, 1987:59-79.

132. Lytle SS, Hall HW. Software, libraries, and the copyright law. Libr J 1985 Jul;110(12):33-9.

133. Walch DB. The circulation of microcomputer software in academic libraries and copyright implications. J Acad Libr 1984 Nov;10(5):262-6.

134. Brooks DT. Copyright and the educational uses of software. Educom Bull 1985 Summer;20(2):6-13.

135. Smith SC. Managing academic software: leadership, law, and logistics for administrators, faculty, and publishers. McKinney, TX: Academic Computing Publications, 1988. (EDUCOM/Academic Computing software initiative monograph series no. 0899-2592).

136. Kahin B. Property and propriety in the digital environment: towards an examination copy license. Educom Bull 1988 Winter;23(4):15-24.

137. Quint B. Connect time. Wilson Libr Bull 1989 Jan;63(5):86-7.

138. Talab RS. Copyright and other legal considerations in patron-use software. Libr Trends 1991 Summer;40(1):85-96.

139. McKirdy PR. Copyright issues for microcomputer collections. In: Intner SS, Hannigan JA, eds. The library microcomputer environment: management issues. Phoenix, AZ: Oryx Press, 1988:96-125.

140. Gasaway, Copyright law in the age of technology, op. cit.

141. Hannigan GG, Brown JF. Managing public access microcomputers in health sciences libraries. Chicago: Medical Library Association, 1990:97.

142. Valauskas EJ. Copyright: know your electronic rights. Libr J 1992 Aug;117(13):40-3.

143. Basic Books, Inc. v. Kinko's Graphics Corp., 758 F.Supp. 1522 (S.D.N.Y. 1991).

144. American Geophysical Union v. Texaco Inc., 802 F.Supp. 1 (S.D.N.Y. 1992).

145. Gasaway LN. Photocopying ruling affects for-profit sector. Bull Amer Soc Inf Sci 1993 Dec/Jan;19(2):11-2.

146. Crews KD. Copyright law, libraries, and universities: overview, recent developments, and future issues. Working paper presented to the Association of Research Libraries, October 1992.

147. Amicus curiae brief for appellant, Association of Research Libraries, et al, American Geophysical Union v. Texaco Inc., 802 F.Supp. 1 (S.D.N.Y. 1992), July 23, 1992.

148. Medical Library Association supports Texaco appeal [news release]. Chicago: Medical Library Association, April 1993.

149. American Geophysical Union v. Texaco Inc., 802 F.Supp. 1 (S.D.N.Y. 1992), aff'd, 1994 U.S. App. LEXIS 30437 (2d Cir., Oct. 28, 1994).

150. Wiant SK, McClure LW. Texaco settles out of court. MLA News 1995 Aug;(277):22-3.

151. Feist Publications, Inc. v. Rural Telephone Service Co., 111 S.Ct. 1282 (1991).

152. Celedonia BH. From copyright to copycat: open season on data. Publish Weekly 1991 Aug 16;238(37):34-5.

153. Hane P. After Feist: feast or famine in the information industry. Database 1991 Oct;14(5):6-7.

154. Funk CJ, Pierceall KS. MLA headquarters and copyright. Bull Med Lib Assoc 1993 Oct;81(4):445-6.

155. Medical Library Association. The copyright law and fair use. Chicago: The Association, November 1994. (Position statement).

156. Medical Library Association. Copyright and lending software. Chicago: The Association, March 1995. (Position statement).

157. Fair use in the electronic age: serving the public interest. Working document. ALAWON 1995 Mar 11;4(22).

158. Nimmer M. Nimmer on copyright. New York: Matthew Bender, 1993.

159. Patterson LR, Lindberg SW. The nature of copyright: a law of users' rights. Athens: University of Georgia Press, 1991.

160. Matheson N. Copyrights and the user's rights: an editorial. Bull Med Libr Assoc 1993 Jul;81(3):330-2.

161. Ibid., 330.

162. Crews, op. cit., 18.

163. Model policy, op. cit.

164. Crews, op. cit, 18.

165. Bennett S. Copyright and innovation in electronic publishing: a commentary. J Acad Libr 1993 May;19(2):87-91.

166. Matheson, op. cit., 330.

167. Sapp G, ed. Access services in libraries: new solutions for collection management. New York: Haworth Press, 1992: xiii.

•

.

2

Access

Valerie L. Su

This chapter focuses on core areas of providing access in health sciences libraries: collection arrangement, circulation systems and services, stacks maintenance, security, and facility management. While Chapter 1, Administration and Organization of Services, covers organization, budgeting, staffing, and training in circulation, as well as access policies and performance measures, this chapter attempts to offer a pragmatic discussion of the operation of a circulation department and the impact of decisions made about procedures, systems, and the physical library. The emphasis is on access from within the building rather than from remote locations. Although these management issues sometimes seem less exciting than those of electronic access, it is these efforts that enable the user to have actual hands-on access to the physical items.

It is important to remember that each library is unique. Different library users have different needs. Different staff will have different approaches. Each library must develop policies and procedures according to its own environment, user needs, collections, facilities, budget, and staff resources. The description of services, policies, and procedures that follows is based on fundamental, generic library principles. The various descriptions are intended as guidelines to be considered in planning access services and must always be evaluated in the library's own context. Although much of the discussion describes larger libraries in order to cover the range of topics, it is hoped that the concepts and basic principles are obvious and applicable to smaller libraries.

Hours of Access

In the physical library, as opposed to the virtual library, access is limited to the hours the library is open. Only when the library is open does the user have full access to the rich resources of the collections and services.

Some small hospital libraries may be staffed only on a part-time basis, but the collection will be accessible up to 24 hours a day. For larger hospital libraries and academic institutions, extensive staffed hours are needed for patient care information needs and for students. The number of hours that academic health sciences libraries are open ranges anywhere from 62 to 168 hours per week [1]. These longer hours usually are shortened during school intersessions and the summer. For most health care environments, provisions are needed for access for emergency patient care situations when the library is closed .

Hours should be kept as regular as possible so that users can easily remember and rely on the schedule. They also should be publicized widely. The library's regular hours should be posted prominently at the entrance of the library, and the schedule should be advertised in publications and descriptions of the library. When the library is not staffed, using an answering machine or voice messaging system to give hours is very helpful. Many libraries have a telephone number for a recorded message concerning hours and other information. Schedules should be planned well in advance to meet the deadlines of the institution's publications. Academic health sciences libraries may need to do this in the spring or summer for the following school year.

When deciding whether to close for a holiday, one should consider whether the students will need to study or whether the hospital and clinics will be open for regular business. A good rule of thumb is that the library should stay open if the users are not taking a holiday. Holiday closings and changes in hours should be publicized well in advance.

Policies and procedures for emergency after-hours access need to be developed and made known to both potential users and security personnel. Instructions need to be kept in an obvious place in the library, either at the entrance or at the circulation desk. They should include the definition and requirements for emergency access (normally an emergency patient care information need), who has the authority to define the emergency (such as the senior health care professional on the clinical service), and how to gain access to the locked library (by contacting security). These instructions should also explain what the security officer needs to do (stay with the person in the library as the information is located, complete a form to document the nature of the emergency entry and the identity of the user, and provide information about any items removed from the library). They should also include information on how to contact library staff for reference service or in case of building emergencies.

Collection Arrangement

Decisions on collection arrangement have a long-lasting, significant impact on both users and staff. Location and organization affect the convenience and success of access to the collection. The librarian should consider how long it takes to retrieve an item and what barriers exist to finding an item by asking such questions as what are the distances, traffic paths, and typical work flow and use patterns.

Since the emphasis is on the most recent information, the health sciences collection is likely to consist of approximately two-thirds journals and one-third monographs. Print is still the focus, but a contemporary collection will also have other media, especially audiovisuals and computer software. Sometimes titles will consist of multimedia, such as books with slides, books with computer disks, and interactive programs with CD-ROM, videodisc, and print. Table 2-1 shows examples of MARC publication formats and media types.

Based on the characteristics of the material itself and the perspective of users and staff, a library may have a number of subcollections that have varying loan periods and different requirements, such as location, access restrictions, shelving arrangements, and type of shelves or storage units. Subcollections add up easily and quickly as size of the total collection and complexity of user needs increase. One academic health sciences library with over 300,000 volumes has approximately 100 unique locations specified in their online public access catalog (OPAC). A reference collection alone might contain locations for periodicals, indexes and abstracts, monographs, ready reference, vertical file, microforms, and telephone books. The need for separate locations must be weighed against the potential confusion in finding items in multiple subcollections.

Libraries arrange material in sequential order. The order may be either alphabetical by title, alphanumerical by classification number, chronological by date, or by accession number. The choice of order may be different for each subcollection but must be consistent within the subcollection.

The majority of health sciences libraries shelve books and journals separately. In an informal survey on the Internet Medical Libraries Discussion List (MEDLIB-L) in February of 1993, 104 academic, hospital, and other libraries responded as to how they arranged their journals. Nearly all, 101 of them, shelved their journals alphabetically by title: either word-by-word of the full title, by keywords following the *List of Journals Indexed in Index Medicus,* or by Cutter numbers within the National Library of Medicine (NLM) W1 classification [2]. Usually the unbound issues of journals are

Table 2-1: MARC Formats and Media Types

FORMATS	Books	Archives/ Manuscripts	Computer Files	Maps	Sound Recordings	Visual Materials	Serials
MEDIA TYPES							
Print	•	•		•			•
Audiocassettes	•	•			•		•
Records					•		
Compact discs					•		
Models						•	
Photographs		•				•	
Videocassettes						•	
Microfilm	•	•					•
Microfiche	•	•					•
CD-ROM	•		•				•
Computer disks		•	•	•			•
Magnetic tapes	•	•	•	•			•

shelved separately. Books are almost always classified by subject. Though any classification scheme can be used, the NLM classification is predominant and best suited for health sciences library collections.

Depending on special needs of a collection or its use, material may be segregated from the main collection. Examples based on type of use are the reference and reserves collections. Reference materials are typically used for quick consultations for factual, specific information. Materials on reserve are normally put in this controlled collection to maximize use and ensure equitable sharing. Certain types of material that suffer a high loss rate or are vulnerable to mutilation are usually placed in a controlled or monitored collection, often the reserves collection. Exam review material, books with fine illustrations, atlases, books on popular or controversial topics, and expensive materials are all high-risk materials.

Other materials which may be grouped in separate locations because of their use or unique organization include archives, rare books, library literature, government documents, consumer health or patient education, and leisure reading. In addition, rare books collections require security and special environmental conditions. Material on a subject, such as history of medicine, may also be kept together.

Some libraries display the most recent issues of journals for current awareness browsing. New books are also often placed on display before being shelved in their proper location.

A decision to divide the collection by publication date may be made for a variety of reasons. A smaller, current collection shortens the distance most users have to walk when gathering material. The more current collection may be kept on the same level as the entrance while the older material is placed further away. In crowded stacks, requiring frequent shifting of the collection, segregation by date may help by limiting the size of the collection to be shifted. Often, space limitations force remote storage of older, less used material. The disadvantages of dividing a collection by publication date, the potential inconvenience and confusion of two locations for one title or one subject, should be weighed carefully against the need.

Libraries often shelve oversize material (thirty centimeters or more in height) together to economize shelf space and to protect the material. Small material may be more easily found and preserved if kept together in special storage units.

Frequency of use, type of use, and user habits may influence the loan period assigned to a subcollection or type of material. Reference material which requires brief consultations and frequently used journals which users prefer to photocopy may be designated noncirculating to ensure availability. For high security titles or CD-ROM discs, on-site circulation procedures may be needed. High-demand textbooks may be put on reserve with limited loan periods, while other monographs may circulate for longer periods. For further discussion on loan periods, refer to Chapter 1.

Circulation Systems

The fundamental principle of circulation services is to provide access to materials in the collections to as many users as possible in an equitable manner. Policies, procedures, and data files must be established to manage these services. For more information on access policies, refer to Chapter 1. This section will discuss the circulation system based on the policies.

The basic objective of circulation control is to keep a record of the lending transaction, so that the library knows who has what item for how long and, when necessary, can take appropriate action to have the material returned. Before a system can do this, the rules or the parameters of the system need to be in place.

The discussion of parameters is applied here to an automated system, but the concepts can be employed for a manual one. Whether a manual or

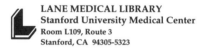

LANE MEDICAL LIBRARY
Stanford University Medical Center
Room L109, Route 3
Stanford, CA 94305-5323

LANE MEDICAL LIBRARY USER APPLICATION
Print legibly and complete both sides of this form

Library ID: 145		Stanford ID:

Name_____   _____ _____   ❏ male
                    Last   First   Middle   ❏ female

Please check the box by the address and phone where you would like your correspondence sent.

❏ Dept./Office Phone: (415)_____-_____   Beeper #:_____   E-mail Account:_____@_____

❏ Dept.:_____ Room #:_____   Mail Code:_____   Rte. #:_____
                                                  (Med Center only)

❏ Local Address:
_____   Home Phone: (___)____-_____
  (Street)

_____   _____   _____
  (City)   (State)   (Zip)

❏ Permanent Address:

_____
  (Street)

_____   _____   _____
  (City)   (State)   (Zip)

The undersigned agrees to abide by Lane Medical Library regulations.
The undersigned agrees that the use of Lane Medical Library's resources and services must be related to the instruction, research, patient care and public welfare goals of Stanford University and Stanford University Medical Center; or for the personal use of the undersigned, who is an eligible member of the Stanford community. The user's library privileges may not be sold or transferred or used in the context of employment by an external business. Use of Lane Medical Library for an external business must be purchased for a fee. Proxy privileges are available to qualified individuals. Library privileges may be revoked for cause at any time.

I give Lane permission to reveal my name to others who need to see the item(s) I have borrowed.   YES___NO_____

Date:_____/_____/19_____   Signature:_____

                         Working Title:_____

OFFICE USE

Time period of library use: From_____/_____/19_____   To_____/_____/19_____

Identification:_____

Pat. Type:	REG	STU	COURAC		Pat. Type
	COURT	UC	OTHER		Pat. Stat.
Verified by:					Pat. Affil.
_____					Dept. Code.

Figure 2-1: User Application Form (Front), Lane Medical Library, Stanford University

CIRCLE ONE AFFILIATION

[M] SU MEDICAL SCHOOL (SUMS)

[H] Stanford University Hospital (SUH)

[C] Lucille Salter Packard Children's
Hospital @ Stanford (LSPCH)

[S] STANFORD UNIV., NON-MED CTR
incl. Hoover, SLAC

[F] Faculty Practice program/Clinic (FPP)

[I] Howard Hughes Med. Inst. (HHMI)

[R] SUL Affiliation
Research Libraries Group in Mtn Vw (RLG)
Ctr. Adv. Study Behav. Sciences (CASBS)
Graduate Theological Union (GTU)
Northern California Cancer Program (NCCP)
Carnegie Institute of Washington
National Bureau of Economic Research(NBER)

[U] University of California (UC)
Reciprocity - Faculty, Acad. staff, residents,
interns, postdoc, grad students

[N] No Stanford Affiliation:
❏ Representing a company or organization
❏ Representing Self

[Z] To be determined

❏ Other (Please describe: _____)
_____
_____

ACCESS ONLY

[Q] SUMS Affiliation
Palo Alto Vet. Admin. Med. Ctr.   (PAVAMC)
Santa Clara Valley Med. Ctr. (SCVMC)
Kaiser - Santa Clara
Research Libraries Group Members (RLG)

CIRCLE ONE CATEGORY

FACULTY

[F] Academic Council

[T] Academic Staff (teaching or research)

[W] Physician Specialist

[V] Acting or Visiting Faculty

[C] Voluntary Clinical Faculty

[E] Emeritus

MEDICAL STAFF

[R] Housestaff Resident/Intern   [I] Visiting Housestaff

[H] Admitting Physician

STUDENT

[S] MD/MSTP   I   II   III   IV

[G] Graduate degree candidate Dept: _____

[D] Post-doc

[K] Visiting Clinical Clerk   [U] Undergraduate

[M] Special Program   [Y] Non-matriculated

[Q] Other (e.g. high school) _____

STAFF

[N] Nurse

[P] Other Healthcare Professional (e.g. dietitian, clinical
social worker, psychologist, speech and hearing
clinician, research pharmacist, etc.) _____

[O] Other Staff _____

OTHER

[A] Stanford Alumnus   [L] Retired Staff

[B] Visitor   [J] Visiting Scholar

[X] Other (check one)
❏ Spouse/Child/Domestic Partner
SU Faculty, Student, Staff: _____
Dept. _____
❏ Director Special (date memo on file) _____

[Z] To Be Determined (Please describe if none
of the above apply: _____)

Figure 2-2: User Application Form (Verso), Lane Medical Library, Stanford University

an automated system is used, parameters for circulation services are required. An automated system simply requires a more rigorous approach and forces the documentation of precise details.

The principal parts of a circulation system are a patron file and a check-out file. An integrated system links the master inventory item file with the patron file and provides the basic functions of check-out (or charge), check-in (or discharge), renewals, holds, recalls, and overdues.

The patron file of registered library users includes sufficient information to identify and contact borrowers, including name, status, one or more addresses, telephone numbers, e-mail address, and expiration date of library privileges. Each person is assigned a unique identification number and codes for various demographic information. For example, a two letter code can identify the institutional affiliation, such as school or department, and the borrower type, such as faculty, student, staff, or visitor. These codes can be used to produce statistical reports on amount of circulation by borrower category. Figure 2-1 is a sample user application form and Figure 2-2 contains examples of user affiliation coding.

In an automated circulation system, each item in the item file carries a unique identification number that is linked to a media type with a loan period and other specific conditions governing the loan. The media type is conceptually a collection as well as a location. Each media type (e.g. book, bound journal) is coded for 1) loan period, including noncirculating; 2) whether the loan period can be overridden; 3) whether renewals are allowed and, if so, the maximum number permitted; 4) whether holds on an item by other users are allowed and, if so, the number permitted and the number of days a hold may remain active; and 5) whether recalls before the due date are allowed. The loan periods and other policy parameters may be varied by borrower category in conjunction with the media type.

A borrower may be blocked from checking out items because of limits specified by the library. Such limits might include the maximum number of items any user or borrower category is allowed to have charged out at any one time; a dollar limit of fines; or a limit of a specified number of overdue items, lost books, overdue recalls, or returned items which cannot be located. Variations or exemptions from blocks may be defined for borrower categories.

Fines may be linked to either the media type or borrower category. The following questions need to be answered. Are fines applied to categories of material or borrowers? What are the fine rates? If there is a grace period, what is the number of days an item may be returned after the due date without having a fine assessed? Is there a fine limit, that is, the maximum amount a borrower may be assessed for an overdue item? Will there be fines for items that have been recalled and not returned? The schedule for the

DATE	ACTION IF OVERDUE ITEM NOT RETURNED OR RENEWED
DD = Due Date	
DD + 7 days	*Send first overdues notice* ⇓
DD + 21 days	*Send second overdues notice; Call borrower* ⇓
DD + 33 days	*Check shelf* ⇓
DD + 34 days	*Add replacement cost to record* ⇓
DD + 35 days	*Send invoice*

Figure 2-3: Overdues Notice Procedure for Items not Returned or Renewed

generation of overdues notices must also be defined. Figure 2-3 provides a sample procedure.

Automation

Circulation systems can be manual, manual with machine-assisted systems which employ devices like credit card charging machines, or automated. A few years ago the big question was whether a library should automate or not. The question now is more likely to be how to automate or how much to automate, or whether to enhance or replace the current system. There are fewer barriers to automation. Microcomputer-based library systems are now reasonably priced, starting as low as a few thousand dollars [3].

Of the 145 academic libraries reporting in the *Annual Statistics of Medical School Libraries in the United States & Canada,* 129 had online catalogs, 117 had automated circulation systems, and 130 provided some sort of online databases or CD-ROMs [4]. This infrastructure supports the call for the use of computer technology in medical information and education in the 1982 Matheson-Cooper report [5] and the 1984 *GPEP Report* [6].

Hospitals have automated their medical records and billing systems, and physicians, nurses, pharmacists, and other health care professionals have become accustomed to automation in their work environment. The Joint

Commission on Accreditation of Healthcare Organizations (JCAHO) 1994 standards incorporated library services within the information management framework [7].

Before discussing automated systems, it should be noted that there are some libraries for which a manual system is still appropriate. The library that can still be well served by a manual system would be one with low circulation and no significant need for management control. Most likely the users must use materials in-house and do not need remote access to information about library holdings. Descriptions of simple circulation systems using book cards, edge-notched cards, and a card system in conjunction with a charging machine are still available [8-10]. For very small libraries that do not need an integrated computer library system, library suppliers have inexpensive circulation control software for both IBM compatible and Macintosh microcomputers.

The main reasons to have an automated circulation system that is linked to an online catalog are convenience, efficiency, and improved management. The ability to have remote access by modem or direct network links—to find out whether the library has a book or journal, whether the title is checked out, and when it is due back—saves the user considerable time. For staff, efficiency is enhanced in basic circulation functions, accounting functions, user registration and maintenance of the patron file, and statistical reports for management decisions and collection development. Tasks can also be performed more accurately and systematically. Some procedures which remain manual are streamlined, such as searching for missing material with a list in call number order generated by the system. Better management information becomes available, such as usage reports by subject area.

Preliminary Steps

Planning for an automated circulation system should include determining the needs of both users and staff, understanding how the library's automation fits into the overall automation and networking plans of the parent institution, and investigating how other libraries have automated. General information is available from books [11-12], articles, and colleagues. The April 1 issue each year of *Library Journal* has a library automation feature [13]. *Library Systems Newsletter* surveys the library automation industry to get an overview of the market and to facilitate comparison among vendors. The results are published annually in the March and April issues [14]. *Library Technology Reports* describes individual systems [15]. The exhibits at annual meetings of library associations are also a good place to obtain information from library automation vendors. Vendors will gladly send demonstration software. Some have prepared information on why and how to automate [16]. As soon as the library has determined what it wants to do, it is important to start building support from administration, the library committee, influential library users, and the institution's systems staff. An analysis of what works well and what doesn't in the current manual procedures should also be undertaken.

Requirements

Each library should make its own list of required and desired circulation functions. Those defined in Appendix A are representative examples to appraise.

Other general requirements to be considered include:

- What other modules are available, e.g. cataloging, acquisitions, serials check-in, authority control? How well do the modules meet the library's specifications?

- What kind of computer or microcomputer is required? Does the system require specific terminals which are available only through the vendor?

- Can the system be on a local area network? Can more than one terminal access the circulation system at a time? How many terminals can be used simultaneously?

- Can users have remote access to the public access catalog from office or home?

- How fast is the system? What size files and number of transactions can the system accommodate? How often does the system have to come down for processing reports or loading data?

- Does the system conform to standards, such as MARCII, NISO, Anglo-American Cataloging Rules, and network and electrical standards?

- What security is provided to prevent accidental or unauthorized modification or destruction of records?

- Are the searching capabilities adequate? Are truncation, Boolean logic, no character limitation for single words, and call number browsing possible?

- Is this system adaptable to health sciences library needs? For example, can it accommodate detailed contact information for users and common circulation needs such as serial volume and single issue check-outs?

- How would the library's system fit in with the institution's overall automation plan? What computer platform(s) are used or supported in the rest of the institution? Would the library's system be compatible with the hospital's information system? In an academic institution where there is a main library and a separate health sciences library, should there be the same library system?
- Last, but not least, what is the price of the system?

The user friendliness of the system is an important element. In circulation departments where staff turnover is relatively high and where student or volunteer help is used, there should be good prompts available on the screen. Documentation and user manuals should be of high quality, and there should be good help screens. The information displayed should be easy to read, and the layout of the template should facilitate quick and easy inputting. It is desirable to be able to do a variety of transactions transparently and to move quickly from one level to another. The library may also wish to be able to customize text and compose or edit help screens and notices.

The reputation of the vendor is also a factor in the decision. How long has the company been in business? How viable are they? How many programmers do they have? How flexible are they in trying to meet their customers' needs? How many other health sciences libraries have bought their system? What kind of training and service do they provide? What is the reputation of their customer service? A reference check with their customers should always be done.

After careful analysis, it is very likely that a single system will not have all the desired features and functions on the list of specifications. It is very expensive for a library to develop its own custom system, and it is not advisable given the number of commercial systems available. There comes a time to be realistic and opt for the best choice available. Once a decision has been made, it will require a high degree of flexibility to incorporate the system and meet the needs and goals of the library.

Implementation

The following is a checklist of steps to undertake while implementing the system:

- Identify everything that has to be done and make a timeline; monitor and readjust the timeline as necessary.

- Learn as much as possible about the system to be installed from vendor demonstrations, documentation, test file, and visits to other library sites which use the system.

- Plan where the terminals or workstations will be located. Order any necessary accessories or furniture.

- Reevaluate circulation policies and procedures and rewrite if necessary.

- Redesign the user registration form so that it matches the patron screen. Develop or revise coding system for user affiliation and status.

- Revise forms and user handouts.

- Involve staff as much as possible in developing new policies, procedures, and forms.

- Do a lot of advertising at different stages of preparation and implementation. Inform as many users as possible by a variety of creative means.

- Develop training exercises for the staff and make sure they have time to put in adequate practice.

- Have a backup procedure to charge and discharge items manually when the system is down. Some libraries have optical character recognition (OCR) numbers printed below the bar codes, not only for equipment flexibility but also for visual identification when a scanner malfunctions or the system is down.

- Determine security procedures, including storing backup system tapes off-site.

- Finally, go online with balloons and fanfare.

Circulation Services

New Book Service

Many library users enjoy browsing through new books received by the library. The more traditional ways of informing users are to display book jackets, to post or distribute a new book list, and to place new books on a new book shelf. Materials on a new book shelf should be well-flagged so that they are reshelved properly for the time they are on display. The shelf should be visible to the circulation staff to deter theft and to facilitate answering questions about circulation procedures.

There are several ways an automated library can disseminate a new book list electronically, such as on the library's bulletin board, by Internet gopher and World Wide Web (WWW) server, by e-mail using a distribution list, or on the "news of the day" of the OPAC.

Ideally, the means of notifying library users of new books and journal subscriptions should be individualized according to a user's specific interests. Although some librarians manage personalized service with manual systems, it is difficult. For those libraries with OPACs, the user probably doesn't need to rely on the library to send or post a list. The user can easily search for new material. Browsing by call number and searching by year are advantageous features for this.

Searches for Missing Material

Libraries should make every effort to assist users in locating materials when they need them. This includes provisions for searching for missing materials. Searches may be initiated by users or by library staff. Many libraries request that users look for an item more than once before a formal search is initiated since items are frequently in use or in the process of being reshelved. Users should be encouraged or assisted in verifying the holdings record and circulation status and in checking such locations as photocopy rooms and sorting areas. Figure 2-4 illustrates the essential procedure and timeline of searching for missing materials. Staff performing the searches need to be trained thoroughly in the use of library systems and in the most likely locations to find materials which are misshelved. Searches should be kept up-to-date, and users systematically informed of ongoing progress and alternative options for obtaining materials. Since material has a tendency to show up or be returned to the library eventually, it is wise not to declare the item lost too soon.

Terminal and Microcomputer Workstation Support

Reference, systems, audiovisual, or separately designated staff may have primary responsibility for support of public terminals, CD-ROM players, and microcomputer workstations. The circulation staff may be requested to help with housekeeping responsibilities such as turning machines off and on, dusting, cleaning the screens, and adding paper and ink cartridges as needed. If evening and weekend reference service is not provided, the circulation staff may need to provide elementary support such as helping users to log in and print.

SEARCH	DATE	ACTION 1	ACTION 2
First	Date Search Requested (DSR)	*Verify: library holdings circulation record not on shelf other possible locations* ⇓	*If found, notify user* ⇓
Second	DSR + 7 days	*Verify: circulation record not on shelf other possible locations* ⇓	*If found, notify user or if not found, ILL option* ⇓
Third	DSR + 21 days (2 weeks after Second)	*Same as above* ⇓	*Notify user* ⇓
Fourth	DSR + 49 days (4 weeks after Third)	*Same as above* ⇓	*If not found, continue searching on a monthly basis* ⇓
Final	(6 months after Fourth)	*Declare item "lost"*	*Order replacement and change cataloging records*

Figure 2-4: Search Procedure

Reserves Collection

The purpose of the reserves collection is to provide immediate and equitable access to material that supports the school curricula, in-service training, and continuing education programs. Most academic health sciences and larger teaching hospital libraries have a reserves collection. Smaller libraries may combine reserves material with the reference collection. There are also some models where the reserves collection is in the media or learning center.

There are two primary categories of material on reserve: permanent or textbook reserves and temporary or class reserves. The principal format of the permanent reserves is books. The class reserves include books, photocopied articles, and copies of old exams. With digital imaging becoming easier to do, some libraries are starting to scan some of the class reserves material which normally would be photocopied and providing access via single workstations or a network. The reserves collection may also include audiovisuals and computer software along with high-loss items such as atlases.

The reserves collection can be organized in a variety of ways depending on the shelving and space limitations of each library. Textbooks on permanent reserve are usually arranged in call number order. Class reserves books can be integrated with textbooks or shelved separately by call number, course, or accession number. Other material such as photocopies can be kept in binders by course number or put into separate envelopes or folders and filed by accession number. These may be kept on the same open shelving as the books or in filing cabinets. It is very important to have the material labeled. "Reserves" tape, wrapped around the top of the spine, works well for permanent reserve items. For temporary reserves, stickers are preferred.

Whatever the organization, access tools are important. A reserves module of the OPAC manages material by course and is linked to the catalog as well as the circulation file; all reserves items are searchable by author, title, course number or name, and professor. For those without a reserves module, at least the books can be in the online or card catalog. In some OPACs a search can be done combining the subject and the location designator for reserves collection. Most libraries find a binder or card file listing class reserves by course number a convenient and easy access tool for students to use and for staff to maintain, with or without automated reserves access.

Whether the reserves collection is an open or closed stack will depend on each library's facility, the size of the collection, and staffing. A closed stack provides maximum control. An open stack reserves collection allows browsing by the user. If in close proximity to, and in view of, the circulation desk, an open stack can function reasonably well. A self-chargeout system helps control an open stack, but it cannot enforce the limited loan period.

The reserves collection is heavily used. Students, house staff, staff, and faculty consult it frequently. Reference librarians consider it an extension to the reference collection. Specialists find the basic textbooks useful when they need to review another field. If the library does not have a consumer health collection, laypersons are referred to the textbooks on reserve.

Reserves is typically a no-growth collection. Collection development policy for the permanent reserves should include the subjects to be represented and to what level, which editions, how many copies, and specifics such as hard cover versus soft cover. It is important to weed and assess the collection at least once a year. Class reserves should be removed after each quarter or semester or when the course is over.

In larger libraries, responsibility for the collection may be shared by circulation and collection development or reference staff. Most often, circu-

To: Medical Course Coordinators

From: [*contact person*]
Lane Medical Library Reserves
L109, MC-5323
e-mail: lanecirc@krypton.stanford
723-4578

Re: Class Reserves Materials

Now is the time to send us a list of course materials you would like put on reserve. If e-mail is not convenient, please call 723-4578 for forms. You will need one form for each course. Please send us your lists before [*date*] as some materials may need to be recalled from patrons, ordered from the publisher or bookstore or borrowed from another library. This process can take up to four weeks since patrons are given the opportunity to finish using the books until their due date.

Include the following information for each course:

BOOKS	Indicate title, author or editor, copyright date and edition.
JOURNALS	Indicate title, volume number, date, pages of article, title of article and author.
REPRINTS or COPIES OF ARTICLES	Please send two copies. Please send materials in folders or binders. No loose pages. Copyright law must be followed.
EXAMS	Please send two or more copies.
PERSONAL MATERIAL	To ensure a safe return to you, please make sure that your name and department phone number appear on each item.
NON-PRINT MATERIALS (videotapes, slides, computer software, etc.)	Please contact [*contact person*] (3-5853, laneflrc@krypton) to place non-print materials on reserve in the learning center.

Feel free to add things to your list as the quarter progresses.

To facilitate access to the class reserves, your lists are kept in an index card file on the reserves counter in the library, filed by course name, and will indicate the location of the reserves items you requested.

At the end of each quarter, these materials will be taken off the reserves shelves and returned to the stacks area of the library. Your personal items will be returned to you or you may send someone to pick them up.

Please call if you have any questions.

Figure 2-5: E-mail Requesting List of Class Reserves Material

lation staff are responsible for contacting the faculty to find out what materials to put on and to take off class reserve and for processing the materials. The circulation staff also have the firsthand knowledge of the extent of use and demand for reserves titles. Collection development or reference librarians are usually responsible for defining the scope and overall collection development and weeding policies of the reserves collection.

Active management of the class reserves is a necessity. Faculty must be kept informed of policies and procedures. When new faculty arrive, a class reserves handout should be included in their library orientation packet. Approximately six weeks before each new quarter or semester, a memorandum should go out to the faculty or course coordinator to request the list of class reserves. See Figure 2-5 for a sample e-mail message.

Copyright considerations are extremely important in the management of the reserves collection. For more information on copyright and reserves, refer to Chapter 1.

Self-Service Photocopying

It is essential that any library have at least one photocopier. Over the past five years, data from the *Annual Statistics of Medical School Libraries in the United States & Canada* show that in-house use of library material is 77% of total library use. The mean number of photocopies in academic health sciences libraries is close to 1.5 million photocopy exposures [17]. The small hospital library is likely to experience a similar percentage of in-house use, but with considerably lower volume of photocopying.

Self-service photocopying in larger libraries may generate significant revenues. Some libraries choose not to own and service the photocopy machines themselves, but rather to contract with vendors. In other cases, the library must follow institution-wide decisions on the selection and operation of photocopy services.

Copier Selection

In choosing a copier, the most important considerations are suitability for anticipated use, reliability, copy quality, preservation features, and repair support. This checklist provides factors which may be important to review.

- **Model.** Library or book copier types have angled edges which allow books to be copied without pressing down on the spines.
- **Ease of use.** This is critical for public copiers.

- **Monthly copy volume.** For an academic health sciences library, a copier that is rated over 100,000 exposures per month should be considered. Durability, or reliability, is the most important quality. Most copiers marketed as library copiers are rated for a volume of less than 100,000 copies per month.

- **Copy speed.** The measure normally given is number of copies per minute. For library book copying, the measure needed for evaluation is how long it takes to make the first copy, i.e. first copy speed.

- **Platens.** The platen is the glass surface on which the item to be copied is placed. A platen with an angled edge allows copying closer to the book spine, with less damage to the binding. The platen should be level with the machine surface. Platen size should accommodate the types of material most often copied. Fixed platens are best; moveable platens are not appropriate for high volume book copying because they increase the risk of tearing and dropping materials and they are slower.

- **Paper tray capacity.** The size should be sufficient to handle the volume of exposures in a day or for reasonable time intervals for paper reloading.

- **Warm-up time.** This can range from one to fifteen minutes.

- **Security.** Lockable internal parts and paper trays are important for public machines.

- **Covers.** These are necessary, but often inconvenient. Flexible hinged covers that can accommodate books versus sheets of paper are preferable. There is at least one machine on the market that does offer a topless feature with an automatic "retina shield."

- **Preservation features.** Copiers with angled edges and support for books prevent damage from books hanging over the edge; heavy journal volumes with weak spines are at particular risk. Tungsten-halogen light units with negligible ultraviolet output reduce destruction of paper and fading of ink caused by ultraviolet light.

- **Coin or copy control features.** These are needed if there is high volume copying by users and cost recovery is required. The copier should be able to be equipped with these items.

- **Options.** Other features which are often on want lists are the ability to have different copy sizes such as letter or legal, multiple copies, sorting and collating, enlargement and reduction ratios, double-sided copying, and single- or multiple-sheet feeders. The needs of the users will determine the final choices. In a setting where the copier also supports the clerical work of staff, the features decided on will be different from those where the majority of copying is high volume journal article copying done by library users. It is important to keep in mind that the more features available, the higher the repair frequency and staff time spent troubleshooting.

Photocopy Operation

Different types of charging mechanisms can be used. Coin- or currency-operated photocopying should be available in most cases. Other mechanisms are needed when there is high volume copying. Some options are machine-readable debit cards, which require card dispensers and add-on value machines; auditrons which can be checked out for counting the number of copies; and computerized accounting systems that log all transactions and generate reports to provide complete accountability for departmental chargeback. The particular needs of the library and its users must be considered, as well as the expense of the systems, including staff time, relative to the advantages.

Copiers create noise, dirt, and considerable heat. If possible, copiers should be kept in air-conditioned rooms, isolated from the collections and study areas, but in close proximity to the collections. Carpeting helps muffle the noise, but it gets dirty quickly when toner is spilled. Also, airborne black toner dust spreads easily twenty to thirty feet from the copiers. Therefore, the floor covering of these rooms should be vinyl, not carpet, for easier cleaning.

Supplemental accessories for a self-service photocopy area are needed to help both users and staff. Items include dollar bill changers, paper recycling bins, staplers, a paper cutter, and a three-hole punch. In addition, adequate book return shelving is crucial.

Copyright warnings are required. For further information on copyright and photocopy services, refer to Chapter 1. Signs may also be needed to inform users how to obtain assistance, about relevant library policies, such as limits on photocopying time, and how to copy without damaging materials.

Services for Persons with Disabilities

In 1990, the Americans with Disabilities Act (ADA) was signed into U.S. law [18]. The ADA requires academic, public, school, and special libraries in the United States to provide equal access to library services to persons with disabilities. The ADA consists of five titles, each addressing a different provision: Title 1, employment; Title 2, public services and transportation;

Title 3, public accommodations and services operated by private entities; Title 4, telecommunications; and Title 5, miscellaneous provisions [19].

Titles 2 and 3 have the most impact on libraries. A library owned or operated by a governmental entity must comply with Title 2; a privately owned library is the subject of Title 3. Essentially, libraries must provide full and equal access for all persons, including those with any disability, to the book or journal stacks, card catalog or online public access catalog, copy machines, computer terminals, media equipment, telephones, study carrels, and other facilities. Some building features required are access ramps, automatic or easy-to-open doors, elevators, wide aisles, and phones at wheelchair level. There must be wheelchair access to copiers, display racks, and shelves. Some workstation and carrel furniture must be usable at wheelchair height. Comprehensive assistance is necessary at both reference and circulation desks. If required, staff must search for, page, and photocopy information. Tailored tours should also be available. Access and assistance should be provided in such a way as to minimize drawing attention to the disability of the person and to allow individual independence where possible.

In terms of removing existing architectural barriers as required by Title 3, legal and architectural counsel should ascertain what is "readily achievable," which according to the ADA means "without much difficulty or expense." Communication aids and services must be provided unless to do so would be an "undue burden."

Copies of the ADA should be available in the institution's human resources department. Several guides to applying the ADA in libraries have been published [20-22]. The Association of Research Libraries (ARL) SPEC Kit 176, *Library Services for Persons with Disabilities,* contains the results of a survey taken of ARL libraries in the spring of 1991 and provides information for planning and implementing services [23].

Stacks Maintenance

Collection Sequencing

The collection should always be shelved so the user reads from left to right. As Figures 2-6 and 2-7 show, the sequence usually goes from shelf to shelf in a section, then from section to section in a range, then from range to range, possibly from a block of ranges to another block, and sometimes from floor to floor. If it is a large collection with a main aisle separating two long blocks of ranges, the sequence usually ribbons or snakes around the ranges on one side of the aisle and then crosses the main aisle and comes

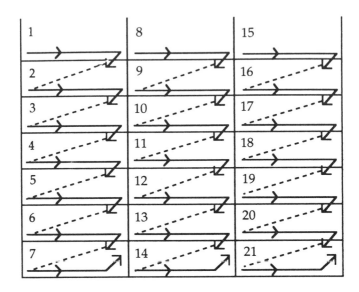

Figure 2-6: Sequencing Shelf to Shelf, Section to Section

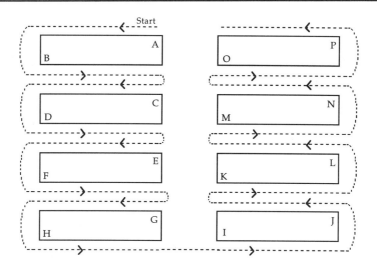

Figure 2-7: Sequencing Range to Range, Block to Block
(Figures by Patty French)

back. In other words, the sequence normally does not cross the main aisle at every range.

A useful exercise in planning the stacks is to draw the sequence flow on the shelving layout, without lifting the pencil from the paper, as the user would face the shelves. The natural starting point should be identified, ideally the closest point to the main entrance. The distance from the last section of one range to the first section of the next range should be kept as short as possible. The flow should be logical and easy for the user to find the next volume in the sequence.

Shelving Equipment

The most common type of shelving for regular purposes is called conventional steel shelving, illustrated in Figure 2-8. Leighton and Weber's revision of Metcalf's space planning classic, *Planning Academic and Research Library Buildings* [24], and Hitt's chapter in the *Handbook of Medical Library Practice* [25] provide comprehensive descriptions of shelving equipment. A summary of basic shelving terminology and measurements is given in Appendix B and Appendix C.

There are also specially designed shelves for specific functions, for different formats and sizes, for special appearances, and for saving space. In a health sciences library, display shelves are most frequently used for current journal issues. Usually the shelves are slanted and the journal issue is fully displayed. With some displays, there is storage behind the shelf to hold the unbound issues of the current volume. Another type allows all issues to be shelved upright and facing out. They are also relatively expensive.

Reference Shelving

Because many of the volumes are large and heavy, shelving for reference periodicals should be no more than six shelves high. If space permits, the fourth shelf from the bottom may be left empty as a consulting shelf. Pull-out consulting shelves can also be useful.

Tables with one to three shelves can accommodate frequently used, oversized indexes and abstracts, such as *Index Medicus*. The shelves need to be at least nine inches deep with a minimum of thirteen inches between shelves. The table can be single-faced, or double-faced with back-to-back shelves in the middle. The tabletops can be flat or sloped.

Reference consulting shelving units, which are three shelves high, can be used for the reference books collection. The tops of the shelving provide

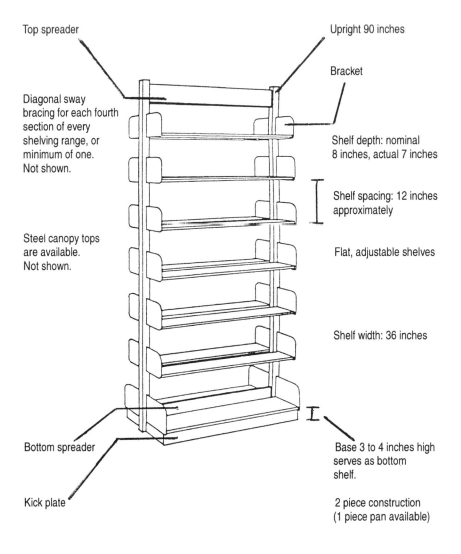

Top spreader

Upright 90 inches

Bracket

Diagonal sway
bracing for each fourth
section of every
shelving range, or
minimum of one.
Not shown.

Shelf depth: nominal
8 inches, actual 7 inches

Shelf spacing: 12 inches
approximately

Steel canopy tops
are available.
Not shown.

Flat, adjustable shelves

Shelf width: 36 inches

Bottom spreader

Base 3 to 4 inches high
serves as bottom
shelf.

Kick plate

2 piece construction
(1 piece pan available)

**Figure 2-8: Conventional Steel Shelving, One Double-Faced
Section.** *(Reproduced with permission of Estey Co., Dickson, Tennessee)*

excellent consulting surfaces. The standard steel shelving can be encased with decorative wood or formica end panels and tops.

Oversize Shelving

Oversize materials require special handling. At least 90% of the volumes in general research and academic collections will be no more than 11 inches high and 97% 13 inches or less [26]. Health sciences collections may have even fewer oversize volumes. Standard shelving with seven shelves in a section will accommodate 11-inch volumes while using only six shelves provides room for volumes up to 13 inches. Oversize materials also require deeper shelves. For a library with few oversize volumes, intershelving or laying the volumes flat on the bottom shelf of a section or on an atlas shelf will be feasible. Shelving the volumes at or near the proper places in the sequence results in a higher success rate for the user in actually finding the items.

For collections with a significant amount of oversize material, it is safer and tidier to shelve them together in one place. The items should be divided into groups by height for better stability, for example up to 13.9 inches high, 14 to 17.9 inches high, and 18 inches and higher. The shelves should be spaced about 15-1/4 inches apart for the 11- to 13.9-inch group and about 20 inches apart for the 14- to 17.9-inch group. A combination of extra long shelving wires and large bookends supports these volumes shelved upright. The 18-inch (and over) material should lie flat on folio or newspaper shelving, where the brackets support the deeper shelf from below. In planning for oversize shelving, the uprights need to be spaced appropriately for the width of the aisle, taking into account the deeper shelves.

Movable Compact Shelving

Compact shelving is becoming popular as a means of saving space. These high-density storage shelving systems are suitable for older or less-used material. They consist of double-faced ranges which are mounted on wheeled carriages. One range is kept stationary, while the other ranges can be moved, either manually or with electric motors, along lateral rails which are installed on the floor perpendicular to the ranges of shelving. The ranges are grouped together with only one aisle per module. An aisle is opened at the place where access is desired by moving the ranges; therefore access is limited to one aisle at a time for each module. Compact shelving systems require a floor load-bearing weight of 300 pounds per square foot. [27].

This author knows that in one busy academic health sciences library, there have been no problems with having journals prior to 1976 on compact shelves. Sam and Major found that "a large shelving installation with seven circulations per hour or more than 600 per week is not too heavily used for satisfactory public access" [28].

Movable compact shelves are safe. Electrical systems have several automatic safety features to prevent ranges from moving if someone is in the aisle. Inoperable electric ranges can usually be cranked open manually. Manually operated systems also have automatic, electrically powered safety features. Signs should be posted to explain how to operate the shelves and where to go for help. If the system does not come with signs, they should be made for each end panel, describing what to do to lock the ranges on either side of the aisle.

It is important to keep the load evenly distributed, with material on both sides of a double-faced range and spread evenly across the range in each section. Materials should be loaded from the bottom and unloaded from the top. A range should not be moved if the load is all on the top shelves and the bottom shelves are empty. Oversize material should not be allowed to hang over the shelves; otherwise, when the aisle closes, they will push into the books on the other side and cause damage to the volumes and shelving. If deeper shelves are needed, the vendor may be able to retrofit the units. The floors and the tracks need to be vacuumed frequently to remove any debris. The mechanisms need periodic checking, and service contracts should be maintained.

Stability

Libraries in earthquake-prone areas need to pay particular attention to shelving stability. Each state will have different requirements. If a significant amount of shelving is to be installed, local building codes or a structural engineer should be consulted. A shelving vendor will also have information.

In the 1989 Loma Prieta 7.1 earthquake, Lane Medical Library at Stanford University had standard library metal shelving with cross or sway bracings, overhead lateral steel channels running from range to range, and non-welded spreader bars at top and bottom of each section. The ranges were anchored to the walls on either end but were not bolted to the floor. Relatively few volumes landed on the floor; however, the force of movement popped the sway bracings, and almost all ranges were out of plumb, leaning from five to thirty degrees. The ranges which were butted to and bolted to walls at one end remained more upright than those which were not. Another library on campus which had free-standing ranges, that is no walls on either side, no overhead lateral steel channels bracing the ranges, and no bolting to the floor, had completely collapsed shelving. All Lane's shelving was replaced with standard metal shelving, with one sway brace for every three sections, welded spreader bars at top and bottom, triangular gusset plates at the base of each upright, and shot-in floor anchors. Overhead lateral steel bracings were not installed. End panels were added more for aesthetics, but these also act as stabilizers, as do closed bases. For areas where stability is a concern, any case shelving or cabinets which are over sixty inches high should be bolted to the floor and/or to the wall. To restrain books from falling off, there are some shelves which have seismic lips and others which use a metal guide bar (one-eighth to one-quarter inch round stock) that normally goes midway on a shelf from one end to the other. The rod swings up when something needs to be removed from the shelf.

Accessories

Since health sciences collections tend to have large, heavy volumes, heavy-duty gauge steel bookends should be used. They should be the appropriate height for the subcollection and have nonskid bases. There is really not a good bookend for oversize, heavy books. Most bookends bend backwards with the weight of the volumes. A flange support in the back which runs directly to the base will help.

Wire book supports attach underneath open style and backstop steel shelves. The wires come in different lengths and widths. One needs a good hand grasp and strength to squeeze the wires together when fitting them into the channels. Care should be taken that the wire ends are properly inserted into the channels before releasing the grip; otherwise it can spring open with force. An under shelf channel can be installed in custom-designed wooden shelves.

Pamphlet boxes or files, often called Princeton files, are used to hold unbound material. The files come in several different heights and are made of plastic, cardboard, or steel. Only cardboard or steel are sturdy enough. It is easier for the user to remove the issue needed if the boxes are only three-sided, with the opening placed facing the aisle.

There is a type of shelving which has slots in both the back and the shelf. Metal plates or dividers fit into the slots. This type of shelving is used for unbound material in place of pamphlet boxes. The material stored on these shelves should not be of a permanent nature nor heavily used because the slots can act as razors against paper and bindings.

Range finders, also known as range label holders or range markers, are 3x5-inch card holders which are placed on both ends of the ranges. The cards indicate the sequence segment of the collection for that range. There are flush-mounted and projected styles. Both kinds work well. The flush-mounted ones can be placed closer to eye level for easier reading as the user walks down the main aisle. The projected holders need to be mounted higher, but the user can see them without turning his or her head. Range finders are available in metal, plastic, or acrylic, and there are magnetic ones for steel end panels.

A variety of accessories is available for messages to inform the user that a title has changed or is in another location. None is perfect. Book-sized blocks tend to be pushed to the back where they fall behind the books and get lost. Plastic label holders, which grip the shelf and also double as book supports, tend to break. Label holders which fit onto the front edge of the shelf have to fit tightly enough or they slip off. For metal shelves, there are magnetic label holders.

Several styles of book trucks will be needed. The flat-shelf book trucks are good for transporting unbound journals and oversize books. The sloping display shelf book trucks, single or double-sided, are best for bound journals and books. The stability of the book truck is important. Some single-sided trucks with three shelves may be unstable when loaded. Wheel size should be examined for stability and for suitability for the type of flooring; larger wheels are needed for carpeted areas. Heavy-duty eighteen gauge steel or sturdy wooden models are best for bound journal volumes.

Book return bins may be placed near reading areas and photocopiers, although they make it more difficult for users to see items which have not been reshelved. The style with a self-adjusting top, i.e. a depressible shelf which lowers as weight is added, helps prevent damage to the books. Infrequently, a thin book might slide through the crack and be caught under the top. The underside should be checked regularly.

Shelving Procedures

Both accuracy and turnaround time in shelving are critical to the user's success in finding the material needed. When a book or journal is not found, the result is that the user may leave without the information, or unnecessary time and effort will be spent verifying holdings, circulation status, and looking for the item. It is in the best interest of all for the library staff to make every reasonable effort to return materials to the shelf in as short a time as possible. Some libraries have a goal of reshelving items within four hours of being picked up or checked in. Backlogs of material waiting to be reshelved should be avoided.

In academic health sciences libraries, approximately 8% of total staff effort is devoted to stacks maintenance. In 1991/92 the mean effort for stacks maintenance was 2.58 FTE (full-time equivalent) or 103.2 hours per week [29]. The workload and the patterns of use will determine how shelving staff are scheduled. In larger libraries, the shelving procedures need to be more complex and rigorous.

Users should be discouraged from reshelving items because they are likely to misshelve. Also, shelving statistics are needed to indicate in-house use. With signs and during orientations and tours, the user can be asked to place items on return shelves and book trucks or to leave them on tables and carrels.

Training and Techniques

It is important to train shelvers well and to check their work. They need to be familiar with work routines, understand the call number and Cutter systems, be able to sort and sequence alphanumerically, remember the locations of all the collections, and know how to respond to questions from users. They also need to be accurate, have good hand and eye coordination, be efficient and neat, and be able to work independently.

The training should include proper methods of lifting and pushing to prevent injuries. They should be encouraged to lift heavy volumes with two hands, not lift too many volumes at one time, use step stools, bend at the knees rather than the waist, and load onto a book truck only the weight that can be pushed comfortably. Shelving for brief periods of time with short breaks is also advisable.

Another important reason for properly shelving volumes is to preserve the life of the collection [30]. All staff should be aware of the importance of the following guidelines.

- Never hook a finger onto the top of a spine to pull a book out.
- Don't use the volume as a wedge. To replace an item, move the bookend or wire sufficiently to allow the volumes to be eased away.
- Keep the volumes perpendicular to the shelf to preserve the binding and spine. To align volumes perpendicular to the shelf, work with a small manageable group at one time. Place one hand perpendicular to the shelf and flat against the lower part of the volume at one end and place the other hand flat against the top of the volume at the other end; gently push the hands towards each other in a gentle rocking motion to straighten the volumes. Use book supports to keep them perpendicular.
- Align the spines of the volumes along the edge of the shelf by using the flat of the hand to either push the volumes from behind or to push back from the front.
- Use two hands to pick up a heavy or oversize volume. Grasp the volume around the spine and support the item from below with the other hand.

- Store oversize volumes flat and limit to stacks of four.

- If oversize volumes are interfiled with regular volumes, store them on their spines. Storing volumes on the fore-edge allows the weight of the pages to pull towards the shelf and the casing to be pulled apart from the spine.

- Avoid letting an oversize volume hang over the edge of a shelf. It can be caught and pulled off the shelf as someone walks by.

- Store thin softcover pamphlets or unbound issues in containers.

- Keep publications of one or two pages in a clip binder.

- Repair damaged volumes before reshelving.

- Do not pack shelves too loosely or too tightly. Report areas of overcrowding.

Shelving Practices

Shelvers should include pickups in their routines. The goal of the pickups is to keep the library tidy for the user and to get material to the sorting shelves and ready for reshelving. In larger libraries a route is defined for comprehensive pickups which includes all subcollections and reading and photocopy areas. Items need to be picked up from tables, carrels, return shelves, and return book trucks. Pickups also have to be made from outside library return boxes. During the comprehensive pickups, any trash from the carrels and tables is collected for disposal, unless housekeeping provides this service. Comprehensive pickups are done at regular times by assigned staff.

The sorting area needs to be located reasonably near the circulation desk, the elevator, the copy center or photocopying machines, and near the collections, to minimize the transporting distances of the used items. Some libraries have sorting shelves on each floor. This works well if the material is used on the same floor as the collection. In libraries where the material is likely to be found on another floor due to the locations of the photocopiers and the reading areas, a single sorting area may work better. The shelves should be marked for rough sorting into subcollections and letters of the alphabet or classification sections. Fine sorting for bound volumes or books can be done from the sorting shelves onto a book truck. The fine sorting of unbound journals may be done more easily at a counter or table. Unbound journal sorting can be done at or near the circulation desk, especially during quiet times.

Shelving statistics serve as an important indicator of the amount of in-house use of library material. Volumes should be counted on the sorted trucks just before shelving, to avoid counting them twice during the process and because items may be removed after they are sorted. Statistics on the number of volumes shelved for each subcollection should be recorded. The statistics are also useful in monitoring the overall workload and the work of individual shelvers. A simple form, kept near the sorting shelves, should include columns for the different subcollections, the date and time period, and sufficient space to write the number for each truck shelved. A card may also be carried by the shelver, with space for initials and assignments for the shift noted by the supervisor.

Since the reference collection receives high use, shelving needs to be done frequently. Due to the usually complex organization of the collection, the shelving is often limited to specially trained circulation staff and supervised or overseen by the reference staff. To help with proper reshelving, the items need to be clearly labeled "Reference" with the specific location, such as index table or reference desk, indicated.

Shelf Reading

A used collection gets out of order. A misshelved book is a lost book. It cannot be helped, but it can be controlled through shelf reading. Shelf reading means to check each classification number or each title on a shelf to make sure the item is in proper sequence. For libraries with collections of several hundred thousand volumes and more, this requires a major staff commitment. Ideally, shelf reading should be given a high priority and shelvers should include periods of shelf reading in their regular routines. Each shelver may be assigned a number of ranges or amount of time to shelf read. A form should be provided to record date, time, and starting and ending points. All subcollections should be shelf read at least once a year. Some heavily used subcollections may need to be read much more frequently. This task is tedious and should be limited to not more than one hour segments. If there is no arrangement with housekeeping to dust the collection, it can be combined with shelf reading to get two necessary tasks done at one time.

Collection Inventories

An inventory is an accounting of every single item in the collection by comparing the items on the shelves to the official record. Inventories are much more time consuming than shelf reading. Although necessary, in practice, they may not be done frequently enough. If a library does not have time to inventory the entire collection, a random sample or a subcollection can be done. For larger collections, another possibility would be to inventory the entire collection over several years. Usually done on a project basis, inventories may be conducted by circulation or technical services staff, or by involving as many staff as possible.

A shelflist, that is a list of all volumes and copies in accurate shelf sequential order, is needed to do an inventory. Some automated systems may not produce a true shelflist, requiring some manipulation of the database by systems staff. The collection should be shelf read immediately before starting the inventory. Efficient procedures should be determined in advance, including how to follow up on items not on the shelf, and supplies obtained. An automated system may generate a shelflist with item status, i.e. on shelf or charged out. After all possibilities have been checked, the item is declared missing and records changed.

The technology exists for doing inventories with automated systems using portable bar code readers. The portable unit is taken to the stacks and the bar code for each item is wanded. A report is generated indicating which items are not on the shelf and whether checked out or not. Hopefully the program shows which items are on the shelf but out of sequence.

Shifting and Moving Collections

Shifting usually is defined as the rearrangement of the collection by readjusting empty space. For example, if the collection has grown too much in one area and the volumes are shelved too tightly, the items in the sections to the right or to the left may need to be shifted further right or left to make room in the tight area. Moving usually implies a bigger project than shifting. Moving can be used to describe relocating a group of items to a noncontiguous area in the library or relocating a collection from one building to another. A library routinely does many shifts or adjustments. These shifts become more frequent, involving more volumes, as the occupied space gets closer to 86% [31]. Major moves are relatively infrequent.

Whether it is shifting or moving, the project needs to be carefully thought through. Even minor shifts need meticulous planning.

- First identify the problem area which has been created, for example, by volumes which are too tightly shelved, a new journal title being added, or a group of books being reclassified.

- Determine how much space is needed to resolve the problem. This requires measuring the existing volumes accurately to the inch and calculating the needed growth space.

- Identify the place in the sequence which needs the additional space, that is, where the items are going to be moved or the area which needs to be spread. Look to the left and right of the sequence to see how and where the extra space can be picked up by redistributing the available empty space. This means measuring the number of inches available in the area to be moved closer together. Try to find the space as close to the section in question as possible. Evaluate carefully to be sure that a problem is not created elsewhere.

In some cases, it may be necessary to remove volumes to a temporary location while work is done on the shelves or the remaining collection is rearranged. It is always desirable to find empty shelves or book trucks to house the volumes temporarily. If necessary, a portion of a collection can be squeezed to accommodate the temporarily displaced volumes, or the volumes can be strip-shelved, which means temporarily storing them on empty top or bottom shelves of another area. Only as a last resort should they be boxed for storage.

Although a shift can be done by one person, it is much better to have two people work together. One person takes the volumes off the shelf and the other places the volumes in correct sequence on the book truck. At the new location, one person takes the volumes off the book truck and the other places them on the shelf. Teams should be used for major moves. One team of two persons takes the volumes off the shelf; another pair puts the volumes on the shelf in the new location. A fifth person is needed to push the book trucks between locations.

Depending on the type and complexity of the move, it may be helpful to mark the shelves and collection. The new sections will be assigned numbers. To indicate the end of a shelf on the book truck, a large piece of paper can be slipped between two volumes with the section number and shelf number.

Whether library staff, professional movers, or volunteers are used, the librarian should supervise the project closely. It is a waste of time and very discouraging to undo moving mistakes, which can happen quickly and involve a large number of volumes. It is critical to reevaluate, remeasure, and readjust frequently as the shift or move progresses. This is especially important for shifts involving more than one range. The final results rarely come out exactly as planned. Throughout a move, users and staff should always be kept informed of the progress and what call numbers or titles have been moved to the new location. The area should also be shelf read after the shift or move.

Shelving Space

The library should keep an inventory of how many linear feet of shelving exist and how many linear feet are occupied. This is important for assessing the availability of growth space and making any necessary plans for remote storage, weeding, or new space.

Before any measurements are made, a map of all the library's shelving should be prepared and ranges numbered. The numbering of the ranges should flow through the library so that each individual subcollection can be defined by a sequence of numbers. Through a spreadsheet, the total linear feet available can be tabulated and calculated. It should include the number of sections, the width of the sections (actual shelf width), and the number of shelves per section for each side of a range. It should then provide calculations for the total number of linear feet per single side of range, the total number of linear feet for the range, the total number of linear feet for the subcollection, the total number of shelves for each width for the entire collection, and the total number of linear feet for the entire collection. The map and spreadsheet should be revised as changes are made.

The best information on occupied linear feet, that is the number of linear feet of shelving the current collection uses, is from actual measurement. This is a time-consuming project, but well worth it if the library is experiencing severe shelf space problems or planning a move to new stacks. An estimate of space needs to be included for items which are checked out at the time of measurement. This estimate can be made by using the average book or journal width for the number of items checked out. An online circulation system can provide the totals; for manual systems, the number of circulating items can be estimated by measuring the inches of check-out cards.

An alternative method of determining occupied linear feet would be to measure the unoccupied or empty space and subtract it from the total available linear feet. A less accurate way to estimate occupied linear feet for a call number range is by using an average number of books per inch of shelflist cards and multiplying by the average width of a book. An automated system might give the number of books in a call number range, which can then be multiplied by the average width of a book.

The occupied linear feet should be maintained on the same spreadsheet as the available linear feet. The spreadsheet should include the beginning and ending call numbers or alphabet and the collection measure in inches for each side of a range. It should then provide calculations for the total occupied linear feet by range, the total occupied linear feet for subcollections and for the entire collection, and the percent occupied linear feet for subcollections and for the entire collection.

The actual measurement of the collection should be done every five years. On an annual basis, the growth of the collection can be estimated by multiplying the number of new journal volumes and number of new books by an average width. Roberts' study gives book width estimates of 1.05-1.11 inches and bound journal estimates of 1.42-1.73 inches [32]. Since journal binding policies affect the width of bound journals, each library should do their own small sample to estimate the average width for their collection.

Before moving a collection onto shelving for the first time, the total available and occupied linear feet should be compared, statistics on growth rate gathered, and decisions made about the number of years of growth space to be allowed and where other empty space should be left. If possible, only six shelves may be used in a section, shelves at the end of ranges left empty and designated for return shelves, and perhaps the fourth shelf in a section left empty for consulting. The same distance between shelves for all sections in a subcollection should be maintained to eliminate the effort needed to change shelf spacing whenever the collection is shifted; it also improves the appearance of the stacks.

Empty space needs to be allocated. If there are known subject areas of more rapid growth, extra space should be allotted to minimize the need for future shifts. The rest of the growth space should be distributed relatively evenly throughout the collection. In the journal collection, volumes of each title will be shelved to the end of the shelf with growth space left after each title and additional space dispersed throughout. In the book collection, empty space should be allowed on each shelf (to accommodate books which may be checked out and for new books) as well as additional space after classification sections and throughout the stacks. Empty shelves in each section or periodic empty sections will provide some insurance when growth rates exceed expectations.

In cases where the existing collection requires less than 40% of the total available space, it should be considered whether it would be better to spread the collection from the beginning to the end of the stack area, or to keep the collection closer together for a few years. The latter option shortens the walking distance for both user and staff initially but will require staff time and user disruption to spread the collection at a later date.

Security

Health sciences libraries can face a variety of security and safety problems. To protect the library's resources and to provide users with as safe an environment as possible, the library must take a number of precautions [33-34]. Having one main entrance and exit, with the circulation staff very visible and close to the door, is by far the best deterrent to thefts as well as other problems. Emergency exits should be attached to an alarm system and plainly marked.

Preventing the unauthorized removal of collection materials is a problem shared by all libraries. Electronic theft detection systems are now common in all sizes of libraries. For these systems, library items need a sensitized tag of the type used in the particular system. There are two kinds of systems. One is a bypass system in which the material stays sensitized, and the library item which is being checked out is passed around the sensing unit or detector. In the full-circulating system, the material is desensitized as it is charged out and then resensitized when it is returned. There are some systems which are integrated with the automated circulation system. A single pass with a bar code reader registers the loan, sets the return date, and deactivates the detection tag for faster, more accurate check-outs. Electronic systems are not foolproof, but they do deter the majority of people. In addition, some valuable collections need to be under lock and key with special provisions for access through staff.

Some libraries that restrict access have a portal monitor who checks identification of users entering and who may also check the belongings of users exiting to see that library materials have been checked out. Since this is labor-intensive, some libraries control entrance by key card or combination lock. This method allows only registered borrowers or primary users into the library. Staff needs to be nearby to handle the exceptional cases.

Mutilation of library material may be minimized by having sufficient photocopiers available, by allowing material to be checked out for copying in departments (where it may be free), and by having enough copies on class reserves. Unfortunately, reasonable lending and access policies will not deter all mutilations.

Audiovisual and microcomputer equipment should be secured with cable and lock kits or anchor pad assemblies or should be locked in cabinets or closets when not in use. Engraving library identification on hardware and furniture helps to deter theft. An inventory of all equipment and furniture should be kept. Bar codes can be used to identify each piece. Making sure that there is someone on duty and in view at all times is an important adjunct to the protection systems.

If cash is collected in payment for library services or fines, it should be kept in a safe or other secure location and regular deposits should be made. Cash theft can be also be minimized by accepting alternative payments, including personal checks, interdepartmental fund transfer forms, and credit cards. Some urban libraries have done away with coin-operated copiers due to the high rate of theft. Equipment such as debit card dispensers and change machines needs to be in sight of staff to minimize theft problems. Standard accounting and auditing procedures also need to be in place.

Library users should be cautioned not to leave belongings unattended. Staff are just as likely to be victimized; they should be reminded to lock their valuables in drawers and not to leave backpacks or purses in view.

Libraries often have to deal with behavioral problems such as acts of aggression, indecent exposure, or disruptive behavior. Staff should be instructed to follow established internal procedures and to report problems to the institution's security department. The institution's emergency number should be kept on the telephone. If the library experiences a lot of problems or is in a high crime area, frequent patrolling of the library by security officers at varying times of day should be requested.

Written closing procedures on how the facility is to be left secure are needed. Both the housekeeping and security departments need to be given a copy of these procedures.

Emergency plans should be reviewed with staff regularly and be a part of orientation for new employees. Staff need to know evacuation procedures and the locations of all emergency exits, fire extinguishers, fire alarms, and other emergency equipment. The lines of authority for making the decision to evacuate should be clearly defined. Staff must make sure all users leave and give assistance to those in need, without placing themselves in danger. The evacuation route and emergency assembly point need to be known. It is essential that all staff meet at the assembly point to be accounted for and to receive further instructions.

It is important for every library to develop a disaster policy to protect resources. Since many excellent publications on disaster planning exist [35-37], detailed information will not be included in this chapter. Emergency supplies suggested in these sources should be assembled, and a manual which includes contact information for assistance and expertise prepared.

Facility Amenities

The importance of making the environment as comfortable and conducive to research and study as possible cannot be discounted. Both functionality and aesthetics are important to consider. For more information on facilities and space planning, there are easy-to-read guides. Freifeld and Masyr's book is for the smaller library [38]. Fraley and Anderson include reading lists in their manual on assessing, allocating, and reorganizing collection and facility space [39]. The Metcalf volume recommended earlier is also a comprehensive source [40].

Furniture and Equipment

There are all types of people with as many different needs and preferences in furniture. The library furniture industry is well aware of this and makes a variety of styles and models available. Even with space and budget constraints, some variety in accommodations should be provided, including carrels, table seating, and lounge seating. Some users want to block out the rest of the world when they work and therefore like the three-sided partitions of carrels. Carrels come singly or attached in various combinations, such as pairs, back-to-back, rows, and pinwheel shapes. Some people may need tables to spread out or share the materials they are consulting. Chairs for carrels and tables and soft upholstered seating offer choice. There is a variety of ready-made furniture designed to accommodate audiovisual and microcomputer equipment which is practical and ergonomically functional. Accessibility for all persons needs to be ensured as discussed in the section on Services for Persons with Disabilities.

Traffic patterns in the library should be considered when deciding where to place the furniture. For studying, most people prefer areas with little traffic. Lounge chairs can be placed in more open, high-traffic areas. If possible, several small group study rooms should also be provided. If there are no tables or carrels near the collection, a few chairs or benches at the end of the ranges permit the consultation of the volumes. Sturdy, slip-resistant step stools should also be placed throughout the stacks.

Use of areas can be somewhat controlled by the type of seating provided. Stools that are reasonably comfortable for short periods may limit other uses of consultation index tables. Chairs should not be provided at public telephones. However, users generally feel quite at home in the library and have no hesitation in moving the furniture around to suit themselves. A staff member should regularly rearrange the furniture according to the library's plan and monitor repair needs.

The general advice for furniture is to buy the sturdiest the budget can permit, because library furniture gets used and abused. There are individuals who dangerously tilt chairs backwards on two legs. Wood veneer on desks, carrels, and tables tends to pop up along the edges and break away.

Special furniture and equipment are needed for the reference collection. Items include index tables, low shelving units which can double as consulting surfaces, large tables for spreading out the indexes and research materials, microcomputer or terminal furniture, quiet printers, a quiet photocopier, lockable storage units for high-loss items, filing cabinets for vertical files, microform reader/printer, and a dictionary stand.

The equipment and furniture needs for a reserve collection are simple. Regular shelving is used. Slotted shelves are useful for pamphlets, folders, and binders. A filing cabinet is best for photocopies. Consulting shelves, tables, and seating for the collection are convenient and keep the material in the area. Also, a photocopier in close proximity is important.

The pros and cons of using book return boxes should be weighed in the light of preservation concerns, user needs and convenience, and staff time to go to the various locations. There are many styles, with advertised protection features against physical damage, weather, fire, and theft. Book return boxes can be placed at the curbside near the library and directly outside the library to provide around-the-clock service. They may also be located in work areas accessible to users. Of course, there should also be a return box within the library, at the circulation counter or desk, ideally with a depressible bottom.

Other Factors

Lighting is also an important consideration. Good lighting in the collection and study and reading areas should be assured. Ideally, there should be some choice of natural and artificial light. If the overhead lighting is very good and there are no shadows cast on reading surfaces, it may be possible to avoid task lighting in carrels. Special attention to lighting and the avoidance of glare is needed where there are computer or video monitors. Energy saving features such as having alternate banks of lighting fixtures on different switches permit the use of half the lights during heat waves or when there is sufficient natural light. For safer, efficient opening and closing of the library, it is preferable to have a master light panel, where all the lights of the library can be controlled. Lights should also be checked routinely for bulb replacement.

Carpeting muffles noise and creates a warmer ambiance than any other flooring. However, it is easier to roll book trucks on linoleum or vinyl. For carpeting where book trucks will be used, a very low, dense pile or tightly twisted yarn without padding may be selected. Uneven textured floors like brick or tile should be avoided. In all cases, the most durable grade of flooring that will be quiet, safe, and easy to clean is desired.

The temperature, humidity, and ventilation of the environment affect the efficiency, productivity, and health of people as well as the longevity of library materials and equipment. Paper does well in a constant environment of sixty to sixty-five degrees Fahrenheit with relative humidity of 50-55% [41]. This standard will have to be balanced with the comfort zone for humans in most areas of the library. High temperature and humidity promote mold and mildew. Humidity below 25% may cause the buildup of static, which can affect electrical equipment. Electrical equipment generates heat and also tends to break down if the room temperature gets too hot. Good ventilation with filters brings in outside air.

Some libraries have an audible public address system or are connected to the hospital overhead paging system. The link to the paging system is a convenience for those needing to answer pages, but the noise can be distracting to other library users. A main advantage of a public address system is to be able to make the library closing and other announcements. With the increased use of paging beeper systems, the need for overhead paging has diminished. At least one house phone is necessary for users to answer their pages. The library may also choose to have public pay phones.

Dust, dirt, and trash are harmful to library material, either directly or indirectly. Food debris and spills lead to damage and insect and rodent infestations. Many libraries have policies prohibiting eating, drinking, or smoking. It is important that the library have a contract or other arrangement with a housekeeping service. There should be a schedule of what housekeeping will clean and when. Provisions need to be made for trash pickup, ongoing dusting of the collection and stacks, and annual cleaning projects such as cleaning and polishing furniture.

Good signage is an art that can be learned. There should be two signage schemes: professional signs for permanent directions, locations, and instructions and staff-made signs or inserts for temporary locations and changing information. Maps are essential, especially for libraries with multiple collections or complex arrangements. The map should be oriented in the same direction as the person reading the map. Stacks should be clearly labeled with directional signs and range finders. Continual reevaluation of how the library is communicating to the user through signs is necessary. The more signs are posted, the less they are seen. The messages should be clear, positive, and friendly.

Conclusion

Several themes have emerged in this chapter. The importance of examining the needs of the user and of planning carefully have been emphasized. Access to the information in the health sciences library is enhanced by an efficient operation, a well-organized facility, and valuable service. However, at the core of circulation services is the staff. They can compensate for compromises which may have been necessary. Their attitude, commitment and courtesy, and knowledgeable and effective job performance are visible to the library's users and will be noted whatever the rest of the users' experience in the library may be. They are the essential ingredient in the library's success.

References

1. Annual statistics of medical school libraries in the United States & Canada, 1992-93. 16th ed. Houston: Association of Academic Health Sciences Library Directors, 1994:27.

2. Lacroix E. Journal shelving. Message to: MEDLIB-L. In MEDLIB-L [Bitnet/Internet listserv]. Start NE, list owner. Buffalo: State University of New York at Buffalo. 1993 Feb 26 [44 lines].

3. Saffady W. Automating the small library. Chicago: American Library Association, 1991.

4. Annual statistics of medical school libraries in the United States & Canada, 1991-92. 15th ed. Houston: Association of Academic Health Sciences Library Directors, 1993:152-3.

5. Matheson NW, Cooper JAD. Academic information in the academic health sciences center: roles for the library in information management. J Med Educ 1982 Oct;57(10 pt.2):1-93.

6. Physicians for the twenty-first century: the GPEP report. Report of the Project Panel on the General Professional Education of the Physician and College Preparation for Medicine. J Med Educ 1984 Nov;59(11 pt.2):1-208.

7. Bradley J. JCAHO tests info management standards. MLA News 1992 Nov/Dec;(250):1-3.

8. Moorman JA. Managing small library collections. Chicago: American Library Association, 1989.

9. Jones CL, Kasses CD. Lending services: circulation policies, procedures, and problems. In: Darling L, Bishop D, Colaianni LA, eds. Handbook of medical library practice. 4th ed. v.1. Chicago: Medical Library Association, 1982: 65-94.

10. Osborne LN. Noncomputerized circulation systems. In: Soper ME, Osborne LN, Zweizig DL. The librarian's thesaurus. Chicago: American Library Association, 1990:153-5.

11. Cohn JM, Kelsey AL, Fiels KM. Planning for automation. New York: Neal-Schuman, 1992.

12. Corbin J. Managing the library automation project. Phoenix, AZ: Oryx Press, 1985.

13. Griffiths JM, Kertis K. Automated system marketplace 1994. Libr J 1994 Apr 1;119(6):50-9.

14. Annual survey of automated library system vendors: integrated, multi-user, multi-function systems running on mainframes, minis, and micros that use a multi-operating system. Libr Sys Newsl 1994 Mar/Apr;14(3/4):17-32.

15. Saffady W. Integrated library systems for minicomputers and mainframes: a vendor study part I. Libr Tech Rep 1994 Jan/Feb;30(1):1-151.

16. Guide to library automation: a step-by-step introduction. Caledonia, MN: Winnebago Software Company, 1992.

17. Annual statistics of medical school libraries in the United States & Canada, 1991-92, op. cit., 86.

18. Americans with disabilities act of 1990, Pub. L. No. 101-336, 104 Stat. 327-378 (1990).

19. Murphy S. The Americans with Disabilities Act. MLA News 1993 Feb; (252):16-7.

20. Foos DD, Pack NC, eds. How libraries must comply with the Americans with Disabilities Act (ADA). Phoenix, AZ: Oryx Press, 1992.

21. Gunde MG. What every librarian should know about the Americans with Disabilities Act. Am Libr 1991 Sept;22(8):806-9.

22. Laurie TD. Libraries' duties to accommodate their patrons under the Americans with Disabilities Act. Libr Admin Manage 1992 Fall;6(4):204-5.

23. Ragsdale KW, comp. Library services for persons with disabilities. Washington, DC: Association of Research Libraries, Office of Management Services, 1991. (SPEC kit 176).

24. Metcalf KD. Planning academic and research library buildings. 2d ed. by Leighton PD, Weber DC. Chicago: American Library Association, 1986.

25. Hitt S. Administration: space planning for health science libraries. In: Darling L, Bishop D, Colaianni LA, eds. Handbook of medical library practice. 4th ed. v. 3. Chicago: Medical Library Association, 1988: 387-463.

26. Metcalf, op. cit., 172.

27. Bright FF. Planning for a movable compact shelving system. Chicago: American Library Association, 1991:7.

28. Sam S, Major JA. Compact shelving of circulation collections. Coll Res Libr News 1993 Jan; 54(1):11-2.

29. Annual statistics of medical school libraries in the United States & Canada, 1991-92, op. cit., 66-78.

30. Lowry MD. Preservation and conservation in the small library. Chicago: American Library Association, 1989.

31. Metcalf, op. cit., 155.

32. Roberts J. Stack capacity in medical and science libraries. Coll Res Libr 1984 Jul;45:306-13.

33. Lincoln AJ. Crime in the library. New York: R. R. Bowker, 1984.

34. Osborne LN. Security. In: Soper ME, Osborne LN, Zweizig DL. The librarian's thesaurus. Chicago: American Library Association, 1990:98-106.

35. Fortson J. Disaster planning and recovery. New York: Neal-Schuman, 1992.

36. Morris J. The library disaster preparedness handbook. Chicago: American Library Association, 1986.

37. Waters P. Procedures for salvage of water-damaged library materials. Washington, DC.: Library of Congress, 1975.

38. Freifeld R, Masyr C. Space planning. Washington, DC: Special Libraries Association, 1991.

39. Fraley RA, Anderson CL. Library space planning. New York: Neal-Schuman, 1990

40. Metcalf, op. cit.

41. Zinn NW. Special collections: history of health science collections, oral history, archives, and manuscripts. In: Darling L, Bishop D, Colaianni LA, eds. Handbook of medical library practice. 4th ed. v. 3. Chicago: Medical Library Association, 1988: 469-572.

3

Interlibrary Loan and Document Delivery

Gretchen Naisawald Arnold and Martha R. Fishel

Interlibrary loan (ILL) and document delivery comprise an important cornerstone of contemporary health sciences library service. For the purpose of this chapter, interlibrary loan service refers to the process of requesting and supplying physical materials library to library. Document delivery represents the transfer of full-text documents in any format (print, page image, electronic) directly to primary users, external individuals, or to organizations without libraries.

This chapter concentrates on the operation of interlibrary loan and document delivery. It examines the influence of developments such as the Regional Medical Library Program and technology-based systems. It details procedures for interlibrary borrowing and lending and document delivery and the current options for automated ILL and document delivery. Chapter 1: Administration and Organization of Services should be consulted for a discussion of organization, budgeting, staffing and training, interlibrary loan policies, and performance measures.

Technology has greatly changed the concept of interlibrary loan and document delivery. One of the earliest changes occurred with the implementation of high quality photocopy systems that allowed libraries to send photocopies of needed items rather than the actual volumes themselves. This procedure ensured that materials were readily available to primary users, and requesters obtained a copy of the item that they could keep. With the advent of computerization and shared cataloging systems such as the Ohio College Library Center (OCLC), now known as the Online Computer Library Center, and the Research Libraries Information Network (RLIN), libraries could quickly and efficiently obtain holdings information for other libraries. The DOCLINE system of the National Library of Medicine (NLM) made another major contribution to interlibrary loan service by providing precise holdings information for journal literature in the health sciences and automating the routing process for requesting documents. Telefacsimile and newer electronic document transmission systems provided faster delivery times, replacing the use of postal or other manual delivery systems with digital technology and high-speed computer networks. The technology behind, and the impact of, automated ILL systems will be discussed in more detail later in this chapter.

Since most libraries and their clientele recognize that no library, no matter how large, can acquire and maintain collections that meet all users' needs, interlibrary loan service provides an important bridge to other library collections. As Horres and Bunting describe in their work, the expanding knowledge base in the health sciences disciplines and the increase in the number and cost of library materials, together with the rapid implementation of modern computer and communication technologies, all encouraged the development of resource sharing systems [1]. Interlibrary loan networks and consortia range from informal agreements among small, local libraries to large-scale national networks supported by sophisticated computer systems.

In the fourth edition of *The Handbook of Medical Library Practice,* Middleton provides an excellent overview of interlibrary loan services; in it he points out that the underlying principle for libraries is mutual benefit [2]. Central to interlibrary loan philosophy is the expectation that each library will maintain a collection that meets its users' basic needs. Beyond this, libraries agree in concept both to lend and borrow materials that are not acquired by the borrowing library because they are peripheral to basic collections, are infrequently needed, or are not collected due to particular constraints such as limited acquisition of foreign language materials. It is natural to assume that the distribution of lending versus borrowing will vary from institution to institution, but reciprocity is fundamental to an effective and efficient system.

Today, the issue is more one of access rather than ownership. As access and delivery systems advance, it becomes increasingly less important that a library actually own an item, but that quick and cost-effective access to the information is possible. The recently revised "National Interlibrary Loan Code" recognizes a shift in the very nature of interlibrary cooperation, with interlibrary borrowing an integral element of collection development rather than an ancillary option [3]. In addition, as document delivery moves into the commercial sector, the role of the library as intermediary for these services becomes less clear and, in some cases, disappears entirely as the user obtains such services directly.

Role of the National Network of Libraries of Medicine

Health sciences libraries are served by their own network, formerly the Regional Medical Library (RML) Program from 1965 to 1991, known today as the National Network of Libraries of Medicine (NN/LM). Bunting's history of the RML Program makes it clear that the value and impact of up-to-date information to the practice of health care became a priority to the federal government in the early 1960s [4]. Bloomquist's 1963 report on the state of medical libraries indicated that dramatic measures were necessary in order for them to meet the increasing demands that would be made by modern health care systems [5]. In 1964, the President's Commission on Heart Disease, Cancer and Stroke, chaired by Michael E. DeBakey, M.D., recommended that the National Library of Medicine be given the mandate to develop and strengthen the nation's medical library system [6]. The resulting congressional legislation in 1965 was the Medical Library Assistance Act (MLAA) which provided support for a variety of library activities [7]. A cornerstone of the MLAA was the formation of a national system of regional medical libraries, which supported the delivery of medical information.

Access to needed information, locally, regionally, and nationally, was a basic underlying concept of the RML Program. Eleven libraries were originally selected to be Regional Medical Libraries, geographically dividing the U.S. into large service areas; the present configuration is eight regions. All the RMLs agreed to provide free interlibrary loans to qualified users within the region, including the provision of free photocopies of materials that were unavailable for loan. The RML Program was by design a hierarchical system with primary access libraries such as hospital libraries at the base, next resource libraries such as academic health sciences libraries, followed by regional libraries, and NLM at the top. In philosophy and practice, requests were directed to local collections first. Those requests unfilled locally were sent to resource libraries or the regional library with NLM as a tertiary resource. This had the effect of keeping most interlibrary loan traffic at the local and regional levels and encouraged the development of better library collections.

Another important contribution was the training and consultation services provided by NLM and the RML Program. By giving network participants at all levels training and expertise in basic interlibrary loan operations, including the use of MEDLINE and DOCLINE, the network could function optimally, and needed information would be available quickly to health care providers. The RML Program was also an early supporter in the development of regional union serial lists which gave libraries, particularly small hospital libraries, precise journal holdings information. Outreach to underserved health professionals, particularly those unaffiliated with health sciences libraries, is a current priority of the NN/LM. Systems such as Grateful Med, a user-friendly front-end search interface for many NLM databases including MEDLINE, and its online document ordering module known as Loansome Doc help provide better access to health care information for this special group and other health professionals.

The NN/LM's impact on health care information delivery has been significant. Most health care practitioners have access to print and electronic resources that provide information necessary for contemporary health care education, patient care, and research that was almost unimaginable thirty years ago. The NN/LM's goal for turnaround of interlibrary loans from resource libraries to borrowing libraries ensures that information will be available to health professionals in a responsive fashion.

Influences on Interlibrary Loan and Document Delivery Service

Today's health care environment is in a constant state of change with new knowledge created every day. Health care has become greatly specialized in nature with clinicians and researchers focusing on increasingly small areas of medicine. As with medicine, nursing has become specialized so that it is not uncommon for nurses to concentrate in particular areas such as pediatrics or geriatrics. Expansion of roles for health care professionals such as respiratory care therapists, occupational therapists, pharmacists, and social workers has created a health care delivery system that is diverse and interdisciplinary.

The literature required to meet the information needs of health care and health care professionals has changed similarly. Some studies indicate that scientific literature grows at the rate of 6% to 7% each year [8]. At this rate, scientific information doubles every ten to fifteen years. The knowledge base supporting medical research has expanded. By analyzing the references in articles in the *New England Journal of Medicine* in 1951 and 1981, Huth found that in 1951, 45% of all references were from ten journals; in 1981, only 14% of the references were supplied by these same journals [9].

An example of the effect of specialization on the health sciences literature is described by Miller and Starr in their analysis of the information explosion in radiology. In 1970, they found 7,072 articles in MEDLINE on radiography and its subspecialties, with general radiography articles, 4,020 or 57%, the largest category. Analysis of the same subject areas in 1985 resulted in 33,945 articles, with only 10,907 or 32% from general radiography, demonstrating that the radiology subspecialties now played a significant role in the development of new knowledge in radiology [10]. It is reasonable to assume that this phenomenon holds true for most medical specialties.

In addition to this growth, existing journals have increased their size. According to Huth, where once the average journal would carry ten articles, it is now common for these same journals to contain twenty to thirty articles [11]. A recent NLM study determined that there was a 56% increase in articles per journal title indexed in the period 1966 to 1985. In 1966 the average *Index Medicus* title contained 67.5 indexed articles, while in 1985 this number had risen to an average of 105.5 articles for each journal title. The number of live serial titles in this subset of NLM's collection also increased 30% in the twenty years [12].

These changes indicate that users and their libraries require access to a greater number of journals, either from their own collections or by borrowing from other libraries, to support their research. Analysis of the interlibrary loan data gathered by the Association of Academic Health Sciences Library Directors (AAHSLD) shows that the number of requests filled by academic health sciences libraries continues to increase. In 1984/85, there were 1,020,592 interlibrary loan requests filled by academic health sciences libraries [13]. In 1992/93 this figure had risen to 1,522,855, representing an increase of approximately 49% [14]. This increase is likely due to the improved access and delivery systems now available to libraries as well as the decreasing ability of libraries to acquire and maintain on-site collections comparable to the expanding knowledge base of the health sciences.

The large indexing and abstracting database search systems such as MEDLINE, formerly the domain of the librarian, became accessible to the health professional with the development and availability of low-cost personal computer equipment and user-friendly search interface software. Cost-effective equivalents of these systems on CD-ROMs or through Grateful Med make them within the financial reach of individuals as well as small libraries.

Quick access to needed information is critical in a health services environment. Decisions affecting the welfare of individuals sometimes hinge on having the latest research in clinical care immediately available. Consequently, great emphasis is placed on fast turnaround times for ILL and document delivery services. Not surprisingly, technology has served this process well. The availability of electronic location information via large computerized systems such as OCLC and DOCLINE has resulted in faster turnaround times for requests, increased traffic on the networks, and changing lending patterns regionally and among different types of libraries. Use of telefacsimile and other new communication and document transmission technologies has provided more responsive document delivery service.

Basic Operations: Policies and Procedures

Interlibrary loan is generally divided into interlibrary borrowing and interlibrary lending. Interlibrary borrowing refers to activities centered around the procurement of materials from other libraries, upon request of a library user, when the materials are not available in the user's local library. Interlibrary lending refers to the other end of this process, which is the supplying of materials from a library's collection to other libraries. Interlibrary loan, both borrowing and lending, as well as document delivery services, are supported by similar procedures and practices.

Several resources will give the librarian new to ILL a solid background and understanding of basic service. The "National Interlibrary Loan Code" defines the purpose and scope of ILL and outlines the fundamental responsibilities of the requesting and supplying libraries [15]. The *Interlibrary Loan Practices Handbook*, published by the American Library Association (ALA), is an excellent source for a detailed practical description of standard interlibrary loan practices and procedures [16]. The *Interlibrary Loan Policies Directory* compiles policy statements for academic, public, and special libraries in the United States and Canada [17]. Many regions, states, and networks have their own interlibrary loan policies and guidelines that should also be referred to as appropriate. DOCLINE users may find the DOCUSER database useful; it provides information on interlibrary loan policies and procedures, telephone numbers, institutional contacts, and library identifiers (LIBIDs) for NN/LM member libraries [18].

Policies governing ILL services differ according to the library's mission and the available resources it has. Every library in some way must ration its resources, be they financial, human, or physical, to ensure that needs of primary users are well served. A detailed discussion of interlibrary loan policies is included in Chapter 1.

In many cases, the size of the library and the typical information needs of its user population will determine what automated interlibrary loan systems it will have available. The efficiency and specificity of the DOC-LINE system, and the fact that the cost for use of the system is subsidized by NLM, make it an attractive candidate for most health sciences libraries. Its use is actively encouraged by local and regional consortia as the preferred method of interlibrary loan, especially for journal articles. Many libraries, including larger academic and hospital libraries, have need for more interdisciplinary materials as well as a broad ranges of formats which cannot be obtained through just one system. Consequently, these libraries are likely to have multiple systems available, such as OCLC and RLIN, as well as DOCLINE. Many smaller libraries which do not use OCLC for cataloging participate in OCLC's Group Access program, giving them the benefit of automatic referral through a larger library, acting as the referral agent, when the request goes beyond the group libraries.

The Association of Research Libraries (ARL) has initiated the North American Interlibrary Loan and Document Delivery (NAILDD) Project, the goal of which is to promote developments that will improve the delivery of library materials to users at costs that are sustainable for libraries. It envisions the integration of information access and delivery mechanisms into online information systems to enable a user to identify, locate, and obtain materials. It assumes seamless interface among systems, supporting institutional and library programs, policies, and practices, and a primary but not exclusive role for the library. Three major objectives of the NAILDD Project include a management system to eliminate paper files and stream-line internal procedures, a financial system to minimize the costs of ILL charging, and linkages between and among local and national systems. Although the project emerges from the research library community, its goals could offer benefits for the library community as a whole [19].

Interlibrary Borrowing

Each library must decide whom it will serve. Since ILL borrowing is a labor-intensive service, it is not uncommon for libraries to limit this service to their primary users. How each library defines a primary user is often governed by its parent institution. In recent years, there has been greater recognition of the needs of unaffiliated users, in particular health professionals working in medically underserved rural and urban areas. Some libraries have relaxed previously more restrictive policies to provide limited services for these individuals. In any case, each library must have a coherent policy on eligibility that can be easily explained by all library staff at service desks.

Many institutions will only borrow certain types of materials. Books and journal articles, usually in the form of photocopies, comprise traditional interlibrary loan service. Some institutions will attempt to borrow audiovisual materials, provided they are available for loan. Many libraries limit their service when it comes to government documents or theses and dissertations. Users needing these items may be referred to appropriate for-profit companies which can supply them.

Most requests are submitted on printed forms that are generally available at library circulation or reference service desks, though increasingly requests may also be submitted electronically or by other means. When possible, it is usually an advantage to have a library staff member quickly review the request at the time the requester submits it so that any omissions can be noted or filled in with correct information; the requester can also be alerted if the item is actually in the collection. Print forms, or printouts of electronic requests, provide a worksheet for interlibrary loan staff and facilitate good record keeping. Information on these forms can be keyed into computerized systems such as DOCLINE or OCLC. The forms themselves are generally incorporated into the unit's working files for records and statistics keeping.

The essential elements of an interlibrary loan request vary slightly with the format of the requested item. For books, these elements include author, title, publisher, place of publication, edition if applicable, any series information, and year of publication. Journal requests should include full title of the journal, author or authors of article, article title, volume and issue number, pages, and date.

Where libraries go to borrow materials can be determined by a variety of issues. Generally, the rule is to exhaust local resources first before moving outside the local area. Often neighboring libraries form informal or formal reciprocal agreements to provide service among participants according to certain guidelines such as next-day service or service without charge. Certain institutions, particularly publicly supported ones, often request from each other first, even though this sometimes means going outside the immediate local area. Eventually, most requests not met locally or through prearranged reciprocal agreements will work their way up through the NN/LM system. Some institutions go outside the traditional library networks and procure documents from commercial sources. Reasons for using these services include copyright compliance since these sources incorporate copyright fees in their charges. Other advantages are the vastness of their resources and fast turnaround times.

Many libraries no longer verify the accuracy of all citations as was once the norm. Quality control efforts to ensure data integrity in most databases and the direct use of these systems by library users have significantly improved the quality of citations. Consequently, many libraries only verify those citations that are incomplete or confusing. When verification is necessary, the availability of journal citation databases such as MEDLINE, HEALTH, and PsycINFO, to mention a few, give interlibrary loan staff excellent and efficient means to verify requests for journal articles. Similarly, the comprehensiveness of systems such as OCLC and NLM's CATLINE database, as well as the particular subject concentrations of systems such as RLIN, make these invaluable resources for quick verifications for monograph citations and serial titles. Retrospective conversion projects for many large academic libraries nationwide also make these systems valuable resources for older materials, although the printed *National Union Catalog* (NUC) or *Science Citation Index* may still be necessary for more obscure, older citations. Most interlibrary loan staff, including clerical staff, can be trained to perform quick and simple searches of appropriate systems and databases for verification of requests. The cost of online charges to perform the searches is generally more than outweighed by the staff costs to verify citations manually through union lists or printed tools. Many libraries encourage users to include printouts of citations they have retrieved from online databases so that the verification is essentially provided for the ILL staff. Libraries without access to online systems such as the ones above must rely on available print tools such as *Index Medicus*, *Abridged Index Medicus*, and any local, regional, or state union lists that are available.

Occasionally there are citations that cannot be verified through any available means. Requesting libraries which choose to send these requests on to other libraries, generally a resource library in the NN/LM, should clearly identify the request as "cannot verify" and include any pertinent additional information such as the journal bibliography in which the citation appeared.

Automated document request systems such as OCLC and DOCLINE assist in the selection of locations of potential lenders to varying degrees as part of their basic operation. OCLC provides holdings information as part of its catalog module, but the requesting library has to manually select the lending institutions. DOCLINE was designed to include precise holdings information and provides a routing table that replicates the typical borrowing patterns of the library. Since holdings information in DOCLINE is item-specific for each participating library, the DOCLINE system can automatically route requests through the system. A detailed discussion of these systems appears later in this chapter, but their implications for basic services are important. Libraries using them do not have to expend staff time predetermining locations as was done in the past, and turnaround time is reduced. Smaller libraries may have to rely on union lists produced by state or local consortia. Since holdings information in DOCLINE only applies to journal information, finding locations for book material without access to systems such as OCLC can be difficult for small institutions. At this point, it may become necessary to rely on cooperative arrangements with larger libraries or programs such as OCLC Group Access.

To minimize transmission times, most libraries prefer to use available electronic systems to send requests to other libraries. Systems such as DOCLINE and OCLC ensure that requests are generally available within the next working day at the lending library. Other technologies such as electronic mail and fax can also offer faster methods of sending requests. All of these technologies depend on having similar systems on the other end. If electronic means are not available, using the traditional ALA interlibrary form and the postal service is the next alternative. Some libraries will agree to take a limited number of requests over the telephone, but this is generally limited to special circumstances such as a patient care emergency.

The daily functions associated with borrowing are listed in Table 3-1. Boucher also contains a detailed explanation of borrowing procedures [20]. Some of the tasks parallel those for lending and can efficiently be performed at the same time. The borrowing library is responsible for ensuring that the requester abides by the conditions of the lending library for borrowed books or other items. Methods for returning borrowed materials are discussed below under Interlibrary Lending.

Copyright issues are an important consideration in interlibrary loan work. Chapter 1 reviews the implications of the Copyright Act and related guidelines for interlibrary loan. It covers the responsibilities of the borrowing library for copyright warning notification, systematic reproduction, copyright representation for requests, and record maintenance for interlibrary borrowing requests.

The ability to check on the status of requests is a basic feature of most electronic document request systems. Library staff at the lending library update requests to indicate that they have been received and when they have been processed. These systems also may indicate whether a request that could not be filled has been referred to another institution. Some libraries also use electronic mail to inquire about the status of their requests.

Those requests that are unfilled require follow-up to ensure that all possible avenues have been explored. Occasionally, a request can be lost or misplaced and needs to be resubmitted. Requests are not filled for a variety of reasons including that the item is missing, at the bindery, lost, or in circulation at the lending library. In some cases, the lending library may determine that the item is too rare or too fragile to be lent to another library or even to be photocopied. The citation may also be faulty.

The decision as to what records are kept is often dictated by the information the library needs to monitor its services both for its own purposes and to report to outside agencies. These can include local consortia, the NN/LM, and state and local agencies. Most academic health sciences libraries report their activities to other groups such as ARL and AAHSLD. In general, most libraries track the number of items they borrow, format of material, number and category of users requesting materials, number of items borrowed from specific institutions, copyright compliance information, number of requests that could not be filled and for what reasons, costs of items, and turnaround times. Many institutions count how requests are

Table 3-1: Interlibrary Borrowing Daily Functions

- Collect requests

- Confirm items not owned by library; verify citations

- Determine copyright compliance

- Ascertain library locations or other sources as needed

- Input requests into online systems (or alternate means of transmitting requests as needed)

- File requests in pending file

- Receive and process filled requests; notify requesters

- Follow up on borrowed materials, including checking due dates, contacting requesters, and seeking renewals as needed

- Prepare borrowed items to be returned for shipping

- Resolve problems

- Perform record keeping activities, including filing forms for completed requests and entering statistics (may be done less often than daily)

---

sent, such as by DOCLINE, OCLC, fax, and mail. Financial data for payments to lending institutions as well as information for billing users need to be maintained.

Records are organized in anticipation of future needs. Records for pending requests are usually filed by user name so that staff can quickly check to determine the status of a particular item or provide a record of all items requested by individual users. These records are also necessary to monitor due dates for materials borrowed and to note any extensions in loan times. Retrospective tracking of requests, by journal or other title, is necessary to ensure that the CONTU guidelines on photocopying for interlibrary loan activities are followed by the borrowing library. These records can be copies of the actual requests themselves or another system such as a database or card file. Specific recommendations for maintenance and retention of records can be found in the ALA "Guidelines: Records of Interlibrary Photocopying Requests" [21]. The section on Policies Concerning the Confidentiality of User Records in Chapter 1 is also relevant.

Most libraries will need to keep financial records even if users are not charged for the service. For those that charge, records arranged by user should be maintained to show status of individual accounts and to follow up on any problems. Similar procedures should be followed for materials obtained for a fee from other libraries to provide accurate records of paid and outstanding accounts. These should be arranged according to lending institutions.

Since interlibrary loan service is an important indicator of library service in general, statistics on it are generally reported to many agencies. Consortia need to monitor ILL traffic to determine if each library is doing its share and to recognize if certain institutions need additional support. Similarly, data are reported to groups such as AAHSLD and the Research Libraries Group (RLG) to track library patterns nationwide or by specific groups of libraries. Internally, interlibrary loan requests contribute valuable information for collection development analysis since they provide concrete information about user needs not met within the current collection, although they must be considered along with other factors.

There are commercial software programs now available to assist in tracking and managing many ILL operations. One such program, QuickDOC, has been specifically designed with DOCLINE libraries in mind. (Further discussion of QuickDOC may be found in the Front-End ILL Systems section of this chapter.) QuickDOC includes functions not only for monitoring requests and report generation, but it also supports such activities as printing forms, uploading requests, and billing [22]. QuickDOC and other ILL management programs can greatly simplify and enhance many ILL activities, although, if several ILL systems are used, it may be necessary to reenter data.

Interlibrary Lending

Each library must determine which institutions it will serve. As a rule, in the spirit of cooperation, most libraries will lend to most other libraries. However, in the interest of conserving their resources, some libraries will serve only other health sciences libraries and decline to serve libraries affiliated with for-profit operations such as corporations or law firms and public or academic libraries. Most academic health sciences libraries serve all types of libraries in the recognition that information needs are today inherently interdisciplinary and require cooperation from all types of libraries.

The preponderance of interlibrary loan is in the form of photocopies that are kept by the individual requester, even though the photocopy is referred to as an "interlibrary loan." The heavy reliance of the health sciences literature on the journal article has encouraged this trend to the point that only in the most unusual circumstances will health sciences libraries lend actual journal volumes. Most libraries lend books and some nonbook materials. Some libraries choose not to lend audiovisual materials because of the delicate nature of the format. Most libraries will not lend materials that are considered rare or particularly valuable. This practice also includes items that are in fragile condition and could be damaged in the shipping process. Materials that are in high demand, on reference or reserve, or very new are usually not lent to outside libraries.

Health sciences libraries recognize that certain requests must receive priority service. Any request associated with a patient care emergency is always allocated the resources it deserves to ensure that the information is available as quickly as possible. Precedence for these requests over others is something that must be a stated service goal. Some libraries handle requests from certain institutions as priority requests. These can include prearranged service commitments such as next-day service among certain institutions. Some libraries may choose to handle all requests from other health sciences libraries ahead of requests from non-health care libraries with the understanding that the time constraints are more pressing in that environment.

Most libraries prefer to receive requests in formal, traditional fashion such as through the electronic networks or on printed ALA forms. Receiving requests in this manner ensures that the requests can fold directly into the work flow of the unit. Paper or hard copies of requests are necessary for taking to the stacks, notes by staff, and record keeping, so requests received through the electronic networks are generally printed onto paper. Some libraries will take rush requests over the telephone or by fax.

The NN/LM standard for interlibrary loan turnaround is four working days, excluding transit times, so health sciences libraries organize their procedures to meet this goal. Large resource libraries with heavy interlibrary loan request loads generally retrieve requests from electronic networks, such as DOCLINE or OCLC, twice a day. Similarly, staff will sometimes pull items for photocopying or mailing twice a day to ensure that backlogs are minimal. All libraries should perform these routines on at least a daily basis so that most requests are acted upon within the next business day. Table 3-2 lists daily lending functions. A more detailed guide to lending procedures is available in Boucher [23].

Libraries send materials in a variety of ways, depending on the time factor, cost, and internal operating procedures of the parent institution. Use of the postal service remains a standard way of sending materials, particularly photocopies. Articles are usually sent at the first class rate but books can be sent library rate or third class. Though considerably less expensive, this service can be slow. Consequently, many libraries use commercial shipping companies to handle their book shipments with faster delivery service considered worth the additional cost. An additional benefit of commercial services is that they often provide pickup of materials at the work site as part of their regular delivery service. Whether using traditional mail or a shipping service, most libraries insure all materials except for

Table 3-2: Interlibrary Lending Daily Functions

- Collect requests (from mail, online systems, other sources)

- Sort requests that cannot be filled for reasons of copyright or cost or time limitations or that require special handling

- Search for call numbers or internal locations and sort for efficient retrieval of materials

- Pull volumes from stacks

- Photocopy items

- Prepare photocopies and volumes and accompanying forms for mailing; check out volumes to be loaned

- Update online systems with request status (or notify or refer manually as needed)

- Prepare invoices if appropriate

- Resolve problems

- Receive and check in returned material; follow up on loans

- Perform record keeping activities, including filing forms and noting statistics (may be done less often than daily)

---

articles so they are protected in case of loss. Fax, now commonly available in most libraries, is another excellent method for sending rush requests in minutes rather than in days. While users sometimes express dissatisfaction with the paper and print quality of some transmissions, new technology is minimizing both of these problems. Using fax for routine service can cause problems for a busy ILL unit with only one machine since equipment tied up with routine transmissions can be unavailable for rush or emergency transmissions.

Systems such as DOCLINE and OCLC have improved referral methods for materials which are not available. Rather than send the request back to the originating library, the library first receiving the request can electronically refer it on to the next library. Smaller libraries without access to union catalog information, either in print or electronic format, may have to rely on larger resource libraries for referral assistance. In these circumstances, resource libraries may receive requests from hospital libraries that are in turn referred to other libraries after appropriate lending locations are identified.

Chapter 1 reviews copyright obligations of lending libraries, including the responsibility to fill only requests bearing a copyright compliance declaration, for maintaining reasonable supervision of interlibrary photocopying, and including a copyright notice on photocopies.

As with interlibrary borrowing, libraries report interlibrary lending activity to a variety of outside agencies. Statistics are normally kept on the number of items they lend, format of material, number of items lent to specific institutions, number of requests that could not be filled and for what reasons, cost of items, and turnaround times. Data on how requests are submitted is also compiled. Basic working files are necessary to track the status of outstanding loans and appropriate due dates, extensions, and overdues. For those libraries that charge for interlibrary loan services, records for accounts outstanding and accounts paid need to be kept, arranged by requesting institution. These records are necessary to follow up on any outstanding accounts and to provide budget information. Management systems which aid in record keeping are discussed above under Interlibrary Borrowing.

More often, materials may be requested to be sent directly to the individual, bypassing the intermediary library. The increasing availability of technology such as fax machines, either in departments or personally owned equipment, makes this a more obvious consideration. However, some libraries are reluctant to encourage this form of direct service for a number of reasons. They prefer to receive requests from libraries so that the requests can be reviewed for accuracy, appropriate records are kept, and any billing and payment procedures can be followed. If there are problems, it is often more efficient to work library-to-library.

Document Delivery Service

In broad terms, document delivery represents the transfer of full-text documents in any format directly to users. For libraries, document delivery service translates to the processes involved in supplying documents from the library's own collection or from other sources. As this is a value-added service, most libraries impose additional charges, but, in a busy health sciences environment, having materials brought directly to the user can be an important timesaving service. (Chapter 4: Fee-Based Services covers the topic of fee-based document delivery service.)

Since most document delivery service represents a significant commitment of staff resources, it is sometimes restricted to primary clientele. Libraries in urban areas with extensive collections may find it financially attractive to offer document delivery services to corporations and businesses in the community. If these services are priced at a higher rate, it may be possible to use the additional financial resources to help offset the overall cost of the service to primary users. To be successful, the service will need to be of high quality with fast turnaround times.

Depending on the level and scope of the library's document delivery program, it may not be possible to serve all users equally. For example, it may be possible to provide fast hand-delivered service only to those users in close proximity to the library. Other primary users working at more remote areas may have to be served through more traditional methods such as mail, interagency mails, or courier services or, more quickly, by fax. These services may impose certain limits such as increased turnaround times and limiting the service to certain formats (e.g., photocopies).

Whether to serve unaffiliated individual users is a question that most libraries must address, particularly those supported with public funds. Traditionally, libraries have been reluctant to do this, preferring to work directly with other libraries. However, with the introduction of NLM's Loansome Doc program as a document request module of Grateful Med, users now have a method of requesting journal articles. From the library's point of view, the Loansome Doc orders appear as a new selection on DOCLINE and provide accurate and precise information. Libraries which do decide to serve unaffiliated users may do so by providing limited service such as photocopying only those materials owned by the library and not offering referrals to other libraries for materials not available. To ensure an equitable use of institutional resources, it is also likely that libraries serving unaffiliated individuals will develop a different fee structure that contains more cost-recovery and eliminates or reduces institutional support of the service.

Libraries which do not choose to serve unaffiliated users can refer these users to a variety of commercial enterprises that provide documents for a fee. For example, PaperChase offers online ordering of documents from MEDLINE by contracting the service to an outside vendor. The cost of obtaining documents from these document delivery services may be greater than the traditional library service, but the turnaround time can be faster.

Most document delivery requests are submitted on forms or as annotated lists of references. Some libraries may choose to take requests over the telephone or through electronic mail systems, but, for reasons explained earlier about the need for paper copies, these requests will be transformed to a standard form or printed. Library service desks are logical sites for distributing forms and accepting requests. Picking up requests directly from users in their offices or place of work is a particularly valuable time-saver that is provided by some libraries. Now that fax machines are so commonplace, many libraries take advantage of them. As integrated library systems and locally mounted journal article database systems become readily available, it is reasonable to expect that users will electronically tag requests that will be routed to the document delivery unit.

How materials are sent will be affected by the format of the material, the geographic location of the user, the available personnel to provide the service, and the time constraints of the users. Some libraries may elect to have only pickup service in the library, while others with more resources may be able to provide actual delivery services to offices, labs, or other workplaces. Libraries may find it practical to build delivery services around existing institutional services such as interagency mail. For service to remote sites, both the postal service and other commercial delivery systems can be considered as alternatives. Again, fax can be used to provide a less labor-intensive but direct delivery service, assuming that users have easy access to equipment. Electronic full-text delivery, an emerging technology available in many larger, academic health sciences libraries, is another alternative to sending actual materials. Though in limited use now, as the technology becomes more affordable, it will provide an attractive service option for other libraries as well.

Document delivery services have important copyright implications. A discussion of copyright and fee-based document delivery is included in Chapter 1.

Automated Interlibrary Loan Systems

Foundations

The automation boom of the 1970s and 1980s may have had a greater effect on the improvement of information transfer and library services than it had on other industries. Because of the nature of the work, many manual processes were easily converted to automated ones once the bibliographic data were in machine-readable format. Automation of multitask library operations such as online catalogs, citation databases, and circulation systems began in earnest in the 1960s. Large academic and research libraries were the first to implement such systems, but at the time most of them were competing for computer resources with others in their institution, many of whom also had high priority needs. Gradually, administrators' recognition of the unique and high-volume demands for computing resources in libraries led to development of independent computer systems for library services and databases. In the early years, the computers provided enhanced access mostly to bibliographic information, but there were usually system limitations on the number of simultaneous users. An added drawback was that computers in the large centers were not linked to one another, so that the work of one library in keypunching, sorting, and storing data was usually only available to users of that system, leading to duplicate efforts at other institutions where the same records were needed.

It hardly seems possible that as recently as the 1970s, shared computing resources and data transfer were a prospect for the future. Librarians were ready when OCLC introduced its shared cataloging services. Very quickly, OCLC's cataloging services were widely used by hundreds of libraries, many of which, skeptical at first, soon saw cost-savings potential to sharing records. This realization provided the first real opportunity for libraries of all sizes and subject areas to use computing services for resource sharing. Though mainframe systems still remained the backbone of most library services, the advent of minicomputers in the mid-1970s generated a booming business creating and selling automated systems and services to libraries. Minicomputer systems offering OPACs, circulation, acquisition, and check-in systems were installed in libraries all over the world. The concept of downloading and uploading data from one system to another became the means by which many institutions created the bibliographic databases necessary for their systems. By the middle to late 1970s, libraries of all sizes were well acquainted with automated systems that could enhance their technical and public services operations. It was at this time that attention turned to automating the increasingly time-consuming tasks associated with interlibrary loan and document delivery.

By the late 1970s, the ease of bibliographic identification and the availability of a wide variety of book catalogs and citation databases created a thirst for equal ease of access to the full text of the materials. Improvements in searching the biomedical literature of MEDLINE or Biological Abstracts through NLM, BIOSIS, BRS, or DIALOG placed further demands on library acquisition and interlibrary loan departments to acquire the needed materials. Automation of interlibrary loan became a priority at several institutions, some of which were already providing automated services of other kinds. Yet, for something so seemingly uncomplicated, the progression of accurate and speedy automated interlibrary loan systems did not move quickly.

Objectives

The objectives of most manual and automated interlibrary loan systems are similar to each other and relatively simple.

- Identify a bibliographic citation.
- Verify the citation.
- Locate a potential lending library.

- Fill out a request form.
- Send the request.
- Track the disposition of the request.

Many of these tasks take time and searching skills. It is also true that the creation and upkeep of much of the necessary data, such as location symbols and individual library holdings, are not so simple. Effective printed and online union lists must be updated frequently, which can translate to redundant and tedious work if the holdings are not tied to an automated acquisitions and receipt processing system. Even if a library is reporting holdings to just one union list group, the process takes care and attention to detail and, depending on the size of the collection and its acquisition activity, can be a time-consuming exercise.

Most of the automated ILL systems which began to be developed in the late 1970s started with basic objectives such as electronic request and referral processes; they have since made some very sophisticated improvements including automated routing using stored holdings data. Regardless of their functionality, all automated ILL systems have two key ingredients: 1) access to bibliographic records and 2) access to machine-readable union list or holdings information stored in a centralized database.

Among the first organizations to have working interlibrary loan systems available were OCLC, NLM, RLIN, and VALNET, the Department of Veterans Affairs Library Network.

OCLC

When OCLC's original ILL subsystem became available in 1979, its design met basic objectives:

- To increase the availability of library resources by speeding loan requests and responses
- To lower the rate in rise of library per-unit costs by reducing staff time needed to verify bibliographic information in the ILL request and to maintain records of ILL transactions
- To furnish patrons and staff with on-line access to a nationwide data base of bibliographic information as well as to information about the status of a particular library's ILL transactions [24].

These objectives and more were met as the OCLC system provided its users with some gratifying features early in the ILL automation process. OCLC users had access to over four million bibliographic records and direct access to the OCLC Online Union Catalog, allowing them to select potential lending institutions whose combined holdings numbered over forty million [25]. An OCLC user could initiate an ILL request from the located bibliographic record, refer the request to as many as five OCLC member libraries, and track the status of the request through the transaction file and the message waiting file. Additionally, the system provided time-triggered actions for ILL requests that were not acted upon within four days, routing those requests to the next potential lender. The savings were in staff time required to track the status of requests and in total elapsed time to fill requests. Often requests are not picked up on a timely basis or filled as quickly as they might be, and time-triggered actions eliminated some delays. The success of the system, however, still placed the burden of holdings identification (linking the correct source with the request) on the borrowing library, which had to manually identify potential lenders.

OCLC's online cataloging and resource sharing system contained over twenty-seven million items, representing forty-five countries and 460 million location listings in 1993 [26]. A document delivery service that links OCLC FirstSearch databases with database producers such as University Microfilm International (UMI) offers article delivery by fax, ILL, mail, and FastDoc, a full-image service that provides automated delivery from scanned collections. In 1994, the FirstSearch service added online access to the full text of one million articles in 1,400 journal titles, supplied by UMI. Articles may be viewed online, or ASCII text can be delivered to an Internet address or local printer [27].

DOCLINE

In 1979, NLM also focused its attention on an automated document request and referral system for health sciences libraries, DOCLINE. What makes DOCLINE unique is that the structure of the system is based on the automatic selection of potential lenders according to machine-readable location and journal holdings information reported to NLM's National Biomedical Serials Holdings Database (SERHOLD). Because 97% of DOCLINE traffic is for journal articles [28], NLM's efforts were concentrated on serials holdings. The collection of this data was a massive cooperative effort among NLM, the Regional Medical Libraries, and individual reporting libraries [29]. Machine-readable data were obtained from about 500 health sciences libraries in 1980/81 and linked to NLM's serials bibliographic database SERLINE by a nine-digit serial title control number (TCN). That number also serves as the bibliographic identifier in the SERHOLD holdings record and is the means by which automatic routing occurs [30]. As of 1994, NLM had acquired more than 1.3 million holdings from over 3,140 libraries, representing over 40,000 journal titles [31]. SERHOLD has expanded over the years to include the holdings of libraries in some of the major bibliographic utilities such as OCLC health sciences libraries and the Medical Library Center of New York. The ongoing effort to maintain and update SERHOLD records remains an enormous task today, but one that continues to be shared among the participating libraries, the RMLs, and NLM, where the data are processed, linked to NLM bibliographic records, and stored for use in DOCLINE. Most holdings records submitted to NLM are in the SERHOLD format, based on the 1980 *ANSI Standard for Serial Holdings Statements at the Summary Level* (Z39.42-1980) and identified in SERHOLD as Level 3, but records in OCLC and standard MARC formats can also be submitted and converted to the SERHOLD format. Regardless of the format of the data, the most important element is their currency. An automated system such as DOCLINE, which makes routing decisions based on the last reported holdings, is only as accurate as the data are reliable. Even today, the majority of reported "routing errors" in DOCLINE are traced to incomplete or inaccurate holdings records.

The building of SERHOLD was key to the successful implementation of DOCLINE, which took place in phases from 1985 to 1987. The automatic routing in DOCLINE is based upon SERHOLD data and a routing table of potential lenders created by each participating library. This table is a hierarchical list of potential borrowing libraries with which the originator has established reciprocal borrowing and lending agreements. The design of NLM's automatic routing feature was based on that used in the Octanet II system in the Midcontinental Region of the NN/LM [32]. A typical DOCLINE routing table has ten cells into which a library can input the LIBIDs of up to twenty libraries, with a maximum of 180 libraries altogether. In the lowest three cells, a library might enter its consortium partners and libraries with free reciprocal service. Cells four through six might be the primary resource libraries and other libraries that charge. Cells seven and eight might be specialized collections and larger university libraries. Cell nine is the RML, and cell ten is always only NLM. Because DOCLINE is linked to MEDLINE, its BACKFILES, and HEALTH, the borrowing library is able to input the unique citation number or perform a search of the SERLINE database for a serial identifier. The routing process starts as soon as a request is entered and the system assigns it a request number. As illustrated in Figure 3-1, the system randomly selects a library in cell one and checks its holdings for the requested title in the SERHOLD database, continuing until a match is found or there are no more libraries to check. This process is repeated in each cell, with NLM being the library of last resort. (Each user can set their own parameters indicating how many libraries to check in each cell before going to the next.) When a potential lender is located, the request is routed to the holding library. When that

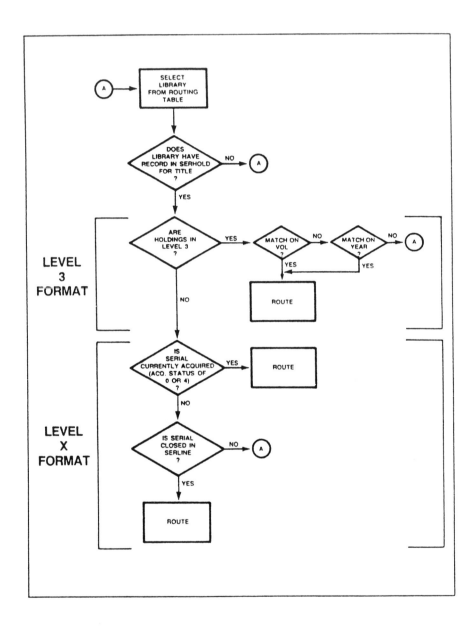

Figure 3-1: Summary of DOCLINE Routing of Journal Requests with SERLINE UIs

lender logs on, they are notified that a request is waiting. Time-triggered actions also exist to assure that requests are acted upon within one day for receipt and within four days for other actions indicating that they are filled, unfilled, or routed on to another library.

VALNET

The VALNET interlibrary loan module was developed by the VA network of hospital libraries in 1984. Many of the VA libraries currently participate in both DOCLINE and VALNET. VALNET was established as a free interlibrary loan system to several VA libraries when NLM still had plans to charge for DOCLINE. As it turned out, the announcement that DOCLINE would be a free service was made in 1985, but by then VALNET was in favored use in the VA system. VALNET uses the Massachusetts General Hospital Utility Multi-Programming System (MUMPS) computer language and includes a complete serials module that permits individual libraries to design and print union lists for local use [33]. The ILL module provides a system-generated prompt similar to that of DOCLINE, then uses an electronic mail system, MAILMAN, to transmit standardized ILL requests. It can track and maintain statistical data for ILL. A proposal to link the VALNET system with DOCLINE is currently under discussion. Ideally, VA libraries will be able to transfer unfilled requests into DOCLINE from VALNET without rekeying data.

Electronic ILL Standards

The need for standardization of library processes and procedures has long been recognized by the National Information Standards Organization (NISO) and the International Standards Organization (ISO). Soon after automated interlibrary loan systems were on the market, work began on creating standards for exchange of ILL data between automated systems. Late in 1991, the ISO formally approved a bibliographic standard for ILL based on the Open Systems Interconnection (OSI) Reference Model. The purpose of this standard or protocol is to permit the exchange of ILL messages between bibliographic institutions that use different computers, systems, and communication services. The protocol formally standardizes four aspects of ILL communications: 1) the number and type of messages exchanged; 2) the data elements contained within the messages; 3) the correct sequence for the communication; and 4) the transfer syntax [34]. This last item is an encoding scheme similar to the tagging method employed in a MARC communications format. Essentially the protocol works by tagging transactions at both ends, from initiation to receipt, processing, shipment, and return. When a transaction is recorded, the library on the other end is automatically notified of the status. As more interlibrary loan systems adapt to the protocol, more libraries will benefit. Transferring requests from one system to another will be possible without rekeying data. Better control over ILL transactions, such as accurate statistics and reporting capabilities, will also result.

The ISO approval of the ILL protocol is key to the unification of library automation services. The National Library of Canada (NLC) developed "test suites" or a collection of test cases covering nearly all applications of the protocol [35], and major Canadian ILL systems have incorporated the protocol. The proponents of this standard believe that the implications are huge and could revolutionize how interlibrary loan systems operate in the near future.

Electronic Mail

In the early 1980s, well before the wholesale acceptance of DOCLINE, many health sciences libraries turned to electronic mail services to meet their basic objectives of fast and efficient ILL service. At that time, the idea that ILL requests could be sent and received quickly, bypassing the time in the mail, was considered to be a great improvement in the process [36]. Today, though most health sciences libraries use automated systems as an access mode for ILL, e-mail still serves a host of health sciences libraries for ILL and other purposes. While its characteristics cannot be fairly compared to those of DOCLINE or other full interlibrary loan systems, e-mail has many attractive features for all kinds of libraries. Essentially, e-mail replaces the telephone as a means of quick communication with another library. It does not require sophisticated equipment, but libraries that use e-mail as a primary means of requesting ILLs are more likely to use microcomputers where they can enter and receive the data offline, store it on the micro, and upload or read messages when they are ready. For libraries where DOCLINE or another ILL system is unavailable, e-mail is a popular, fast, and inexpensive method of sending requests. E-mail systems are easy to use and have at least one distinct advantage over DOCLINE: the messaging capability. Many libraries that have moved to use of DOCLINE for request and referral retain one of the e-mail services for sending messages to other libraries. It should come as no surprise that message topics frequently concern resolution of interlibrary loan problems.

Front-End ILL Systems

Users with modern high-speed equipment expect equally rapid response from the systems they access. While DOCLINE's internal processing time is very fast (seconds to route a request through the massive amount of data in SERHOLD), it takes almost two minutes to complete a request online using the DOCLINE prompts and high-speed data entry. If a mistake is made, it must be caught before the final entry in the input sequence is completed, or the request is sent and must be canceled. In the late 1980s, in an effort to provide faster and more user-friendly management of DOC-LINE's services, Jay Daly of Beth Israel Hospital in Boston created a microcomputer-based front-end to DOCLINE called QuickDOC. This innovative program allows the user to enter interlibrary loan requests offline, resulting in much faster data entry. Users of QuickDOC are not constrained by system operation hours or slower response during peak periods on the NLM computer, nor can they get logged off if they leave the workstation unattended. The requests are validated upon entry, stored in batch, and uploaded to DOCLINE when the user is ready. QuickDOC also offers features that DOCLINE does not yet have, such as a billing module and a completely integrated ILL management system especially useful to the smaller library [37]. With so much emphasis on microcomputer technology, it is likely that NLM will move in the direction of a microcomputer-based system with future enhancements to DOCLINE.

Loansome Doc

The Grateful Med program, introduced in 1986, was designed to make searching NLM's MEDLARS family of databases easier for the health professional. It was evident that Grateful Med users, while satisfied with performing their own searches and retrieving citations, were eager to have a fast way of getting to the full text. Without full-text online databases at NLM, display and downloading of the text could not be achieved. Instead, NLM introduced a document ordering feature called Loansome Doc in 1991. (For further discussion of Loansome Doc, refer to Chapter 5: Future Trends.) Loansome Doc provides a valuable link between the Grateful Med user and the user's health sciences library, and, if necessary, the resources of other health sciences libraries, including NLM. The registration process and ordering steps are simple. Each Loansome Doc user registers with a library for service. That library either provides the documents directly or transfers requests into DOCLINE on behalf of the user [38]. To order a document, a user tags the citations retrieved from a Grateful Med search. From an action screen (Figure 3-2), the user can edit the order list, select a

```
+----------------------------------------------+
| LOANSOME DOC CONFIGURATION SCREEN |
+----------------------------------------------+
Use the ↑↓ keys to move among the various selections shown.  <Home=HELP>
Press the End key to save your ordering information.  <Esc=Cancel>

Delivery Method: Mail Fax Pickup

Delivery Address
    First Name: JUDY            Last Name: JONES
    Organization: ST. MARY'S HOSPITAL
Street Address: 842 MAIN ST.
       City: GREENVILLE
      State: NY Zip: 12882 - 1234
Phone Number: 518 - 555 - 5501 EXT
  Fax Number: 518 - 555 - 3384 EXT

Ordering Library ID: 12345Y    Document Ordering: On Off

Fill orders using additional libraries if necessary? Yes No

+----------------------------------------------------------------------+
| Press <Ins> to toggle the Delivery Method...                         |
+----------------------------------------------------------------------+
```

Figure 3-2: Loansome Doc Configuration Screen

delivery method, and send the list to the MEDLARS order file. The NLM computer then transfers the orders to the user's library using DOCLINE. The library receives the request, fills it, updates the record, and sends the material to the individual user. The status of all orders is updated daily on the NLM computer and can be checked by the individual using the loan status feature of Loansome Doc.

From the libraries' point of view, Loansome Doc citations are accurate, legible, uniform, and are retrieved in one batch for efficient processing. However, despite NLM's promotion of Loansome Doc and its successful pilot period, many libraries were at first reluctant to accept the principle of the system. There were concerns that libraries would be bypassed in the process if a user could order documents directly, and some were worried that they would be inundated with requests. Such concerns have not become reality, but it is the reason that some libraries do not participate.

From the user viewpoint, the system is convenient and efficient. They can order documents any time of the day or night from their home or office and have them mailed, faxed, or ready for pickup. It is clear from numerous comments that users who previously had little or no direct access to libraries are thrilled with their new capabilities. It is equally clear that many of those very same users lose their enthusiasm when they realize that they must pay for the documents provided under the service. Costs vary according to fees established by Loansome Doc libraries, but generally ranged between $6.00 to $10.00 each in 1994. For this reason, presumably, Loansome Doc use has remained low, averaging about 540 requests per day in 1994 [39]. However, the concept of remote access and the ability to order documents with the stroke of a key have kept Loansome Doc in high standing.

As good as many of these front-end systems are, quick access to the full document is what matters most. In the Loansome Doc system, the processes involved in document delivery at the library do not change. When a request is received, it must be taken to the shelf, and the item has to be pulled, photocopied, and either placed in the mail, left for pickup, or faxed. All that has been accomplished is that the user gets in on the requesting process, and the request gets quickly to a source. More and more efforts are now focused on automating the document delivery end of the ILL process. As Jackson noted:

While the "front end" of the ILL process, which includes verifying, locating, requesting and confirming, has been greatly enhanced, the "tail end" of the ILL process has yet to enjoy similar dramatic improvements. The fulfillment and document delivery elements must be the next major challenge for ILL librarians to conquer [40].

Automated Document Delivery Systems

High-Speed Computer Networks

The 1980s spawned a tremendous growth in high-speed computer networks and, with them, a whole new set of acronyms and technical jargon with which most librarians have by now become familiar. It is the development of these networks that has given document delivery systems a hearty boost. In the earlier part of the decade, such networks were in use within academic centers, but by the end of the decade, the National Science Foundation (NSF) had developed a link among several large supercomputing centers, providing researchers and educators with immediate access to the work of their colleagues. This interconnecting gave way to what is now called the Internet, a large "network of networks." These networks communicate through a set of protocols for sending and receiving data called TCP/IP, which stands for Transmission Control Protocol/Internet Protocol. Today nearly all U. S. universities and most government and private organizations are linked through the Internet. Currently, the basic functions of the NSF network and regional connecting networks are in the process of being transferred to commercial regional service providers, with obvious implications for the transfer of costs for many users.

The NSF also has the lead role in developing the National Research and Education Network (NREN), a highly sophisticated system expected to supersede the Internet. With the passage of the High Performance Computing Act in 1991 [41], libraries have an active role to play in assuring that the appropriate researchers and educators have access to the electronic information they need through the NREN.

For libraries and their users, the greatest impact of the Internet is the wide range of library catalogs, publications, and document delivery services available. The user can search a catalog and in some cases request or reserve an item. Many of the newer image-based full-text document delivery systems also make use of the Internet as a means of document transmission.

One of the fastest growing enterprises in the 1990s is group-specific discussion lists, available to subscribers over the Internet. Discussion lists of specific interest to health sciences librarians cover a wide range of topics and include MEDLIB-L, PACS-L (Public Access Computer Systems discussion list), and ILL-L (Interlibrary Loan discussion list), among a current list of about fifty others. Some of the discussion lists, which are generated by users of commercially available integrated library systems or document delivery services, provide a forum for exchange of information among subscribers.

Telefacsimile

Telefacsimile systems have been in existence since the early 1960s, when experiments were in progress at the University of California, Los Angeles. Progress in the technology has made the use of fax machines commonplace in the 1990s. For many information seekers, this availability means that access to full-text documents is no more than a phone call away. Braid observes:

> The concept of facsimile lends itself to document delivery applications. Instead of photocopying pages from a journal and posting them to the user, thereby introducing delays from one to several days, the same pages can be scanned, transmitted, and printed on the user's premises in seconds [42].

Recent advances in the speed of transmission, improvements in the quality of the copy, and the development of machines that have increased memory for storing and sending documents at off-peak phone rates have contributed to the widespread use of fax for both document request and delivery purposes. DOCLINE network statistics for fiscal year 1994 showed that just over 37,000 requests specified delivery of articles by fax. While this was only 1% of the over 2.8 million requests entered into DOCLINE that year, it is important to note that, at the time, less than half of DOCLINE's libraries indicated they were willing to provide on-demand fax service [43].

Telefacsimile machines come in grades, called Groups I, II, III, and IV, which determine the quality of transmission and technical capabilities of the machine, including the vertical and horizontal resolution, transmission speeds, transmission protocols, error controls, and paper size. Currently, Group III machines, with the ability to scan, store, and copy in one step, dominate the market. With Group III machines, a library can scan and store about fifty articles a day and transmit them at night when telecommunications costs are lower. Group IV machines with resolutions of up to 400 dots per inch and speeds of 64,000 bits per second (sending a page in fifteen seconds) are favored for storage and sending where fax is a primary mode of document delivery. However, Group IV machines also have major disadvantages. They cannot use normal telephone networks as Group III machines can, requiring instead a high-speed digital network to which very few libraries have access, and problems of incompatibility with other less sophisticated machines have limited their use as a document delivery service. Cost is another issue because Group IV machines come with a much higher price tag that most libraries cannot afford. Additionally, of all the criteria needed for a document delivery system, the most important is that it be reliable [44]. Fax machines still have too many scanning problems and transmission interruptions to be deemed 100% reliable. Consequently, at this time, the majority of libraries offering fax ILL service still do so primarily for rush or emergency requests.

While it is clear that the technological advances in fax will bring faster and better quality service to many requesters, it is also true that, by itself, it is simply a method of document transmission, a replacement for making a photocopy and mailing it. With all of the competing combined search, retrieval, and delivery systems on the market, fax cannot be called a document delivery system.

Advances in Technology-Based Delivery Systems

Though many are still in their infancy, major advances have been made in document delivery systems from library to library and from library or information source to an individual user. The availability of high-speed communication networks and telefacsimile services are largely responsible. It should be noted that it was not for lack of thought or planning that electronic document delivery systems did not keep pace with the request and referral systems. In fact, much of the technology in use today in delivery systems is not brand new, nor is the idea that it would be desirable, efficient, and maybe even cost-effective to supply documents in electronic form rather than continue the process of mass photocopying and delivery of paper copies. What is new are the refinements to the technology, innovative uses, and the perseverance of a few individuals and organizations. There have been a few systems that have come and gone in the past twelve years; others have had fitful starts and stops. The British Library Document Supply Centre (BLDSC) has experimented with several systems, usually named for Greek gods. Artemis was the first full-scale digitized system which operated under Euronet's telecommunications system. Then came Apollo, using the European Communication Satellite system. In the case of these two systems, cost and limitations in the telecommunications contributed to their demise [45].

The natural evolution for some automated interlibrary loan systems has been to full-fledged document delivery systems. The challenge for developers has been to link the improved access methods with a delivery system that provides what the user wants. In the last few years, several prototype systems have emerged, and a few of them have become successful commercial operations. Some of these systems are telecommunications-based, but the disc-based CD-ROM services were the first to establish a niche in the marketplace.

ADONIS

ADONIS (Article Delivery Over Networked Information System) was the first experiment in supplying full-text documents on CD-ROM. The pilot project, conceived by Elsevier Science Publishers and BLDSC, was provoked by the argument from publishers that photocopying was damaging their print subscription revenue. Armed with evidence from a survey that showed that biomedical articles less than three years old were requested most often, BLDSC approached other publishers to participate in further study, with the lure of a potential commercial document supply service pending on the outcome. The original plan to use optical discs became costly and cumbersome, so it was with great enthusiasm and anticipation that the project turned to CD-ROM digital discs in 1985. CD-ROM discs have many advantages over electronic storage of data, allowing for storage of larger amounts of information at much lower costs [46]. Ultimately, a consortium of ten publishers joined a trial document delivery service to major international document supply centers during 1987/88, which involved the scanning and storing of two years of issues of 219 journals on CD-ROM [47-48]. Now, each week over 600 journals published by the ADONIS consortium are indexed at Excerpta Medica and stored in machine-readable format. The full-text material and a tape of the index data are sent to a scanning facility. Later, the index data and scanned image data are merged, and weekly master discs are produced and distributed to the participating document centers. Articles can be retrieved by access points including author, title, or the unique ADONIS number assigned at the indexing stage. The ADONIS workstations were enhanced by the addition of a multidisc jukebox, eliminating the need to juggle the growing numbers of discs and greatly improving the speed of access to articles [49].

ADONIS was the first successful system for storage and retrieval of full-text articles from CD-ROM, and it marked the first alliance of commercial and noncommercial organizations in a cooperative research and development project in the area of scientific communication. (For further discussion of ADONIS, refer to Chapter 5.) Also of consequence was that ADONIS addressed the copyright issue with publishers. Each time an article is copied it is recorded, enabling publishers to collect a copyright fee, though there are some who argue that the system does not take into account fair use. Preservation and collection maintenance of the printed materials are no longer issues for the titles in the collection, though preservation of CD-ROM is a new area of concern. Binding costs are eliminated, as are costs associated with shelving, book repair, or microfilming. Some tests have shown that retrieval and printing from ADONIS workstations produces savings of up to 50% when compared to the costs of conventional storage, location, retrieval, and photocopying of physical items [50]. Above all else, the item is always available. On the downside, the arrangement with the libraries is a lease agreement, which means that, after all the investment, a library does not actually own the collection.

Ariel

The Ariel system, new in 1991 from RLG, promotes itself as the document delivery system for users of the Internet. Ariel is microcomputer software, available in both Windows and DOS versions, which must be installed at both the requesting and delivering institutions. With the Ariel system, users can scan, store, transmit, and print any text, including photographs, charts, and other graphics, some of which do not transmit well by telefacsimile. Ariel offers high-resolution images printed on regular paper at 300 dots per inch (DPI). The Ariel system can store documents either permanently or selectively. Through a combination of the Ariel software and PC hardware, documents are transmitted over the Internet. An Ariel request is sent on the RLIN ILL System, DOCLINE, or any other electronic messaging system. An ILL request from RLIN can be linked to the Internet address of the recipient's Ariel workstation. An Ariel user has three choices for document disposition: send and delete, send and retain, or print locally [51]. Because document delivery is over the Internet, the cost of delivery is presently less than that of mail or fax. However, some Ariel libraries find that they incur additional costs on labor since it is often the case that a book or bound journal must be photocopied before it is scanned.

Romulus

In 1992, the Canada Institute for Scientific and Technical Information (CISTI) and the NLC announced a product called Romulus, which combines CD-ROM and telecommunications software to enable the user to search union lists on a personal computer from CD-ROM, then dial up and download ILL requests or cataloging records. By 1994, the database contained more than 200,000 records and the holdings of sixty libraries. Advantages to using the Romulus system are that staff can search and create orders offline, then send during off-peak hours to CISTI and NLC via the Internet. Requests sent this way are subject to discount rates, less than orders by telephone, fax, or e-mail. Users find that Romulus is a convenient tool for collection development analysis, and any user can download the data as a union list product [52].

SAIL

An experimental electronic document storage, retrieval, and delivery system called SAIL (System for Automated Interlibrary Loan) was tested at NLM in 1991/92 and used to scan and deliver a small set of journals on a pilot basis. Motivated by the increasing burden on NLM in servicing interlibrary loans in the traditional way, staff of NLM's Lister Hill National Center for Biomedical Communications designed a prototype system consisting of a network of PC-based workstations. An analysis of the interlibrary loan requests during fiscal year 1989 showed that the majority were for titles that had been recently selected for indexing in *Index Medicus* or one of the special nursing, dental, or health lists. A search of SERHOLD revealed that most of these titles were so far held by very few network libraries. Based on this data, forty-four journals were chosen to be scanned and stored in bitmapped images on optical discs. An NLM SERHOLD record was created for each of the titles, indicating it was held in the electronic library. Each scanned article was linked by the MEDLINE unique identifier (UI) to SERLINE and DOCLINE. When a DOCLINE request came in to NLM from the network, the system checked the holdings of the SAIL titles first and, if a match was found for the year and volume requested, routed the request to the SAIL workstation. All other requests were directed to the ILL department for routine processing. What made SAIL different from other electronic document delivery systems was that the requester did not know beforehand that the request might be filled by the electronic library, nor could requests be deliberately routed to SAIL by libraries that simply wanted a document quickly. Requests received by SAIL were automatically processed and printed or, if requested, faxed back immediately, never touched by human hands. The majority of the human intervention was concentrated at the input or document conversion stage which included scanning, quality control, indexing, and archiving of the images. The output processes included document search, retrieval, and transmission. About 120 printed pages, or sixty pages by fax, could be handled per hour. In 1992, an extensive analysis conducted on the SAIL system revealed that the model was not cost-effective, since the major component of the costs were for conversion of the articles into bitmapped images, and most of the articles were not requested during the period. It is anticipated that NLM will continue to use SAIL only to fill requests for materials for which NLM has permission to scan and which are likely to be heavily requested, such as *Clinical Alerts* [53].

Commercial Document Delivery Services

No discussion is complete without mention of the plethora of commercial vendors that have stepped into the document delivery arena just at the point when many libraries were facing difficult decisions about how to cut back collections and increase document delivery services. Beginning in the 1970s, operations such UMI, the Institute for Scientific Information (ISI), and Chemical Abstracts Service were pioneers in commercial document delivery. Now they have many competitors seeking to serve the increasing demands of individuals and institutions. Commercial suppliers can be categorized as one of two kinds: those that make use of a specific existing collection, and those that specialize in finding and supplying documents from a variety of sources, often called information brokers [54]. What generally separates these information providers from traditional library document delivery is that original material is never part of the arrangement. Whether or not the material is retrieved from library collections, and much of it is, what is delivered are photocopies or image reproductions by electronic delivery or telefacsimile transmission. Examples of commercial document providers that use specific existing collections include ISI, whose Genuine Article service supplies photocopies or original "tear-sheets" from the 8,000 scientific journals used in ISI's indexes, online databases, and current contents services, and UMI's Article Clearinghouse, which similarly offers access to article copies from over 10,000 periodicals, usually the same titles that are available on microfilm. The UMI Clearinghouse can be accessed by mail, a variety of electronic mail systems, fax, or their own Articall phone service. The UnCover system is an example of another solution to the intensifying demand for journal literature by a successful commercial document delivery service.

UnCover

UnCover was developed by CARL Systems in 1988 and purchased by Readmore, a subsidiary of Blackwell North America, in 1993. (For further discussion of UnCover, refer to Chapter 5.) The principle of document delivery with UnCover is to create an article index and table of contents database, scan articles upon request, and store them on optical disc for later use. This method is different from ADONIS and the SAIL experiment where whole journals are selected to be scanned, based upon analyzed use criteria. Access to the UnCover system is by the Internet, and it provides article-level access to the journal collections of contributor libraries, currently in California, Colorado, Hawaii, Iowa, and Maryland. The UnCover database is created by CARL systems staff as a byproduct of serials check-in, making it possible to create records at the same time the journals are received. All issues are then forwarded to the holding libraries within twenty-four hours of receipt, so that by the time the library has the issue, the article-level indexing is available in the online catalog. The searcher can retrieve articles by author, keywords, subject, or by browsing an entire journal. UnCover is directly linked to the CARL serials control, so receipt data is available. In the early 1990s, a document delivery component was introduced (originally named UnCover2), allowing users to order any article in the UnCover database. Staff at the contributing libraries retrieve copies of the requested articles, optically scan them, and transmit the images to the central computer in Denver and to a bank of fax servers. This computer handles the fax transmission to the number in the order [55]. Currently, virtually all UnCover documents are transmitted to the requestor by fax. The rationale is that more libraries have fax machines than high-tech machines that can receive digital images, but the real reason is that there are lingering copyright implications to making images and transferring them over the Internet. With the publisher's permission, sometimes a copy of the image is stored in UnCover so that the next request can be filled immediately without intervention. Copyright royalties are tracked, and users can charge their requests to a credit card or establish a deposit account. There is a standard article charge plus a variable copyright fee. In the fall of 1994, the system carried the tables of contents, article citations, and abstracts in 20,000 unique titles [56].

Information Brokers

Full-service suppliers, known more commonly as information brokers, have carved out a big piece of the business of document delivery. A 1993 international directory lists 1,372 entries for information brokers, including libraries, which will perform reference and document delivery for a fee [57]. The work of these companies essentially mirrors those tasks involved in library interlibrary loan. Typically, information brokers offer retrieval of all kinds of publications with fulfillment time ranging from twenty-four hours to two weeks. Ordering procedures vary, but most companies accept document orders by telephone, mail, fax, electronic mail, or telex. Rates vary as well, but usually include a basic per item fee and a per page fee. Additional charges are imposed for rush service.

This type of service, however, can sometimes come into direct conflict with the on-site services and interlibrary loan operations of libraries where the information brokers do their work. At the national libraries including NLM, as well as at many large academic libraries, information brokers spend their days pulling or requesting material from the open or closed stacks and photocopying at the public copiers, creating a conflict with the needs of others using the library facilities. The result is that the libraries end up providing priority service to clients who use information brokers and commercial services rather than to libraries and their users. The physical presence of information brokers has made it necessary for some libraries to implement restrictions on on-site access.

A 1990 study at NLM showed that 2% of on-site users were requesting more than 50% of the material [58]. One of the chief concerns was that material brought to the reading room was not available to be photocopied for interlibrary loan. Additionally, the photocopy machines in the general reading room were constantly occupied by information brokers. This, coupled with the consideration of wear and tear on the collection, resulted in the implementation of a policy restricting the number of requests any one user can submit to twelve daily or 150 annually. In recognition of the needs of the individuals requesting materials through information brokers, the library also implemented a special Information Broker Stack Service, offering a higher volume of service in exchange for a registry of the employees of each information broker working in the reading room. The results of this policy change have been reduced numbers of requests at the desk, down 16% in fiscal year 1992, but greatly increased use of NLM's copyright-cleared Overnight Photocopy Service. NLM offers twenty-four hour turnaround for requests submitted before 3:00 p.m. Many information brokers have found that this service meets their needs, while maintaining their profit margin.

At NLM and many large academic libraries, conflicts with information brokers still exist. The issue is not one of competition for the client, but rather competition for the libraries' services. Most health sciences libraries pride themselves on their responsiveness of service in reference and inter-library loan. DOCLINE figures for 1994 indicated that 94% of all requests are filled, most within four days. On an individual basis, that may not be good enough for some clients whose patent or discovery is dependent on the needed research, and this is why information brokers provide a valuable service.

Individual users and corporate clients are also no longer the mainstays of the commercial document suppliers. Some libraries are finding that it is cost-effective to use document suppliers in place of traditional interlibrary loan and instead of using their own staff [59]. As Kennedy points out:

> In spite of important philosophical differences passed on to librarians
> by the nature of their organizations (academic, government, public or
> corporate), there are signs that the lines separating ILL and commer-
> cial document delivery services are beginning to blur [60].

As evidence, many of the clients of commercial suppliers such as UMI, DIALOG, or OCLC are libraries which use the services of information brokers to fulfill their document delivery needs.

Impact of Automated ILL and Document Delivery Systems

Speed of Service

Speed of service is perhaps the most obvious reason most libraries move to an electronic ILL or document delivery system, though not always the first objective. Eliminating time in the mail alone saves each request minimally two to three days between the time a request is generated to when it is received at the holding library. A system such as DOCLINE, which selects the potential lender, saves additional time by eliminating the manual checking of union lists for holdings, by improving the accuracy of matching requests with libraries, and by automatically referring requests which cannot be filled. Delivery method also clearly affects turnaround. If documents are mailed back, no improvement will be seen in delivery time, but fax transmission or CD-ROM based full-text systems can greatly enhance speed. High-capacity optical storage devices and improved telecommunications systems, such as the Internet, also have an effect on time required for delivery. Other factors include the type of computer or terminal and baud rate. Before automated systems, the turnaround for an ILL was often two to three weeks. Network standards for resource libraries in the NN/LM in 1994 are 75% filled within four days.

Volume of Use

Even before some of the existing automated ILL systems were in place, the prognosticators went to work, pouring over trends in interlibrary loan patterns. Most concluded that widespread use of automated ILL systems would increase interlibrary loan traffic. However, predictions of this type are difficult, because one must take into account the exponential growth of interlibrary loan that would have taken place regardless of the state of automation in ILL. Access to bibliographic databases is already prevalent, creating a high demand for full text. More and more libraries are facing budget cutbacks requiring them to reduce the number of journal subscriptions and buy fewer books. The growth of ILL probably has almost as much to do with the volume of available information as the fact that automation makes it easier to send a request.

Prior to the first release of the OCLC ILL subsystem in 1979, Kilgour conducted a comparative study of the impact of participation in an online catalog on the volume of interlibrary loan of books. His conclusion was that participation in an online catalog would significantly increase ILL and that smaller libraries would see a proportionately higher increase [61]. Similarly, DOCLINE use statistics show a dramatic increase in the overall volume of ILL requests in the network, but the system is designed in a way to prevent an uneven increase to any one library. Properly established routing tables should parallel established routing patterns. If the request goes all through the routing table, selecting libraries at random, and does not find a match, then it is sent to NLM.

As a case in point, the Michigan Health Sciences Libraries Association (MHSLA) studied the impact of DOCLINE on the volume and pattern of ILL traffic among basic unit health sciences libraries in Michigan. The expectation was that the adoption of DOCLINE would significantly increase the volume of ILL borrowing and lending by these units and would change more of them from net borrowers to net lenders. However, after examining six years' worth of ILL statistics comparing predicted increases based on existing trends to actual increases, they concluded that the small deviations could not be attributed to DOCLINE [62].

The overall impact of DOCLINE on the volume of network traffic can be clearly measured. In FY 1987, the total number of requests entered into DOCLINE from the 1,432 participating libraries in the network was 788,105 [63]. Seven years later, in FY 1994, over 2.8 million requests were routed through DOCLINE, an increase of over 250%. The number of participating libraries also rose to 2,671, an 87% increase [64]. The volume of requests received at NLM has risen proportionately. NLM received 192,559 requests from all sources in 1987 [65]. In FY 1994, it received 283,397 requests through DOCLINE [66]. NLM still receives only 10% of all network DOCLINE requests.

Ease of Use

Any automated ILL system must be easy to use. Systems such as OCLC, RLIN, VALNET, and DOCLINE have a series of menus and system prompts which guide the user through the necessary steps. For the most part, the system should be self-explanatory after initial training. Accompanying manuals should be necessary only for reminding the user how a particular feature works. The ILL requesting process has been simplified and streamlined to the point that many libraries can have lower level staff doing much of the input and receipt processing. In addition, no library can afford to have a citation or full-text document delivery system available to users that requires constant instruction on its use by library staff.

Fill Rates

Interlibrary loan fill rates are inexorably linked to document availability. A library could be using the fastest and most efficient ILL system, but, if the item is not on the shelf when a request comes in, the loan cannot be filled. Every library is familiar with the most common reasons for not filling requests: items may be on loan, missing, or at the bindery, or citations may be incorrect. Electronic storage of full text is possibly the one solution to make certain that an item is always available. While CD-ROM products are often expensive, they provide more assurance for the accessibility of material. Fill rates are one of the biggest selling points of some of the new digitized storage systems such as UnCover. Articles stored permanently will surely boost fill rates for frequently requested materials, and a system that automatically verifies requests can minimize problems with citations.

System Features and Adaptability

Most ILL and document delivery packages have a variety of attractive management features. DOCLINE statistics, for example, include both summary and detailed lender and borrower statistics on a quarterly basis. An additional feature with DOCLINE is an annual list for each participant that shows which other libraries have included a library in their routing table. This feature serves as a control for inappropriate routing. Many libraries also make use of the annual ranked list of serial titles requested as an aid in collection development decisions. Furthermore, some ILL systems, such as QuickDOC, have an automated accounting system, a valuable addition to any interlibrary loan system, large or small.

Costs

Any cost savings are usually assumed to be in staff time for functions such as the requesting process, the internal processing of the requests, and the sending or transmission of the requested material. This assumption is made because the system usually takes care of the verification process, the requests are uniform, legible, and accurate, and depending on the storage system, the material is always available. Some additional staff costs, however, may have to be allocated to creating and updating union list data and to the use of multiple systems. While labor costs may be reduced, equipment costs and telecommunications charges can increase. If a library goes to a commercial system, document delivery charges often increase; depending on the service, article costs can easily range from $5.00 to $20.00 each [67]. An examination of the costs of ILL and document delivery, including the costs of automated systems, would track the following factors.

Staff costs. The 1993 ARL/RLG study found that staff costs account for 77% of the cost for ILL borrowing and lending [68]. These are the salaries and fringe benefits which can be attributed to all physical and intellectual aspects of ILL activity, including any contract labor costs. Since it is not uncommon to have the same staff performing aspects of borrowing, lending, and document delivery, it is useful to have some estimate of the percentage of each staff member's time that is devoted to each activity. It is also important to consider the administrative personnel costs of the service that are incurred outside the unit itself. These activities include setting policies, working with national and local consortia, identifying and incorporating new technologies that improve service, and maintaining overall quality assurance for the service.

Equipment. ILL and document delivery services require a variety of equipment for which operational costs should be tracked. Typical equipment needed includes photocopiers, microfilm reader/printers, computers, and fax machines. Since equipment is often leased, the cost per year should be prorated and, if necessary, percentages of use for each activity estimated. Costs of maintenance contracts or actual maintenance charges should be included to give an accurate picture as well.

Online searching. Costs for using the various online systems, both for verification of requests and for sending and receiving requests, need to be included. As more libraries have access to locally mounted databases such as MEDLINE, actual online connect charges to verify citations will be significantly reduced. Currently, NLM underwrites the costs for DOCLINE users, making this an extremely cost-effective system. Other systems such as OCLC do have fees for interlibrary loan system use.

Transmission costs. Costs to send materials include postal fees, commercial shipping costs, insurance, and supplies for packaging materials. Since electronic transfer of materials is becoming more commonplace, costs associated with the use of fax, including equipment and telecommunications costs, should be calculated as well. Systems that utilize the Internet, such as Ariel, have reduced telecommunications costs to date.

Supplies. No operation can run without routine supplies. These include general office supplies, forms, and materials necessary for the operation of the equipment such as toner, special paper, and printer supplies. Boucher lists minimum and recommended additional supplies needed by borrowing and lending libraries [69].

Collection. Costs which would be incurred whether the services existed or not, such as those to develop and maintain the collection, are generally not included. While no one can dispute the fact that ILL and document delivery services can cause wear and tear on the library's collection, these costs, for the most part, are hard to document and therefore are seldom included in the cost of the overall service.

How a library decides to financially support its interlibrary loan service and document delivery programs depends on a number of key factors including the overall financial picture of the library and its parent organization, the particular philosophy of the library's administration towards these services, the prevailing practices of other similar libraries in the region, the volume and demand for the services, and the availability of resources, especially human resources. Further discussion of determining costs and policies for charging is included in Chapter 1 and Chapter 4.

In reviewing the impact of automation on interlibrary loan and document delivery services, it is certain that the systems that exist have made a tremendous difference in information transfer in the last decade. The level of expectation has increased to assume that a very high level of service, accuracy, and immediacy are attainable and at a reasonable cost. It is unlikely that expectations will be reduced in the coming years. Future trends point to an ever-increasing demand for information delivery, and the programs, systems, and services that can meet these demands will flourish.

References

1. Horres MM, Bunting A. Interlibrary cooperation among health science libraries. In: Darling L, Bishop D, Colaianni LA, eds. Handbook of medical library practice. 4th ed. v.3. Chicago: Medical Library Association, 1988:177-219.

2. Middleton DR. Lending services: interlibrary loan/document delivery. In: Darling L, Bishop D, Colaianni LA, eds. Handbook of medical library practice. 4th ed. v.1. Chicago: Medical Library Association, 1982:95-136.

3. National interlibrary loan code for the United States, 1993. RQ 1994 Summer;33(4):477-9.

4. Bunting A. The nation's health information network: history of the Regional Medical Library Program, 1965-1985. Bull Med Libr Assoc 1987 July;75(Suppl 3):1-62.

5. Bloomquist H. The status and needs of medical school libraries in the United States. J Med Educ 1963 Mar;38(3):145-63.

6. U.S. President's Commission on Heart Disease, Cancer and Stroke. Report to the President: a national program to conquer heart disease, cancer and stroke. 2 v. Washington, DC: U.S. Government Printing Office, 1964/5.

7. Medical library assistance act of 1965, Pub. L. No. 89-291, 79 Stat. 1059 (1965).

8. Price DS. The development and structure of the biomedical literature. In: Warren KS, ed. Coping with the biomedical literature: a primer for the scientist and the clinician. New York: Praeger, 1981:3-30.

9. Huth EJ. The hypertrophy of modern medicine and the handling of medical information. Trans Am Clin Climatol Assoc 1983;95:170-5.

10. Miller JDR, Starr L. Information explosion in radiology. Can Assoc Radiol J 1988 Mar;39(1):33-6.

11. Huth EJ. The information explosion. Bull N Y Acad Med 1989 Jul/Aug;65(6):647-61.

12. Humphreys BL, McCutcheon DE. Growth patterns in the National Library of Medicine's serials collection and in Index Medicus journals, 1966-1985. Bull Med Libr Assoc 1994 Jan;82(1):18-24.

13. Annual statistics of medical school libraries in the United States & Canada, 1984-85. 8th ed. Houston: Association of Academic Health Sciences Library Directors 1986:76.

14. Annual statistics of medical school libraries in the United States & Canada, 1992-93. 16th ed. Houston: Association of Academic Health Sciences Library Directors, 1994:29.

15. National interlibrary loan code, op. cit.

16. Boucher V. Interlibrary loan practices handbook. 2nd ed. Chicago: American Library Association. In press.

17. Morris LR, Morris SC. Interlibrary loan policies directory. 5th ed. New York: Neal-Schuman, 1995.

18. News from the NN/LM. MAC Messages 1994 Jul/Aug;(46):7.

19. North American Interlibrary Loan & Document Delivery Project: overview & vision. Washington, DC: Association of Research Libraries, January 1994.

20. Boucher, op. cit.

21. Guidelines: records of interlibrary photocopying requests. Appendix P. In: Boucher V. Interlibrary loan practices handbook. Chicago: American Library Association, 1984:174.

22. Divens B. Streamlining DOCLINE: the QuickDOC software: a review. J Interlibr Loan Inf Supply 1993;3(4):13-7.

23. Boucher, op. cit.

24. Jacob ME. A national interlibrary loan network: the OCLC approach. Bull Am Soc Inf Sci 1979 Jun;5(5):24-5.

25. Mitchell J. OCLC interlending and document supply services; a review of current developments. Interlending Doc Supply 1993;21(1):7-12.

26. Ibid., 7.

27. FirstSearch upgrade provides online access to documents [news release]. Dublin, OH: OCLC, November 1994.

28. Lacroix EM. Interlibrary loan in U.S. health sciences libraries: journal article use. Bull Med Libr Assoc 1994 Oct;82(4):363-8.

29. Humphreys BL. NLM's national biomedical holdings data base: progress report. NLM News 1981 May;36(5):1-3.

30. Willmering WJ, Fishel MR, McCutcheon DE. SERHOLD: evolution of the national biomedical serials holdings database. Ser Rev 1988;14(1/2):7-13.

31. National Library of Medicine Library Operations monthly report. September 1994.

32. Dutcher GA. DOCLINE: a national automated interlibrary loan request routing and referral system. Inf Tech Libr 1989 Dec;8(4):359-70.

33. Department of Veterans Affairs. VALNET fact sheet. May 1992.

34. Turner F. Interlibrary loan protocol: an international standard for electronic messaging - part 2. J Interlibr Loan Inf Supply 1990;1(2):13-25.

35. Ibid., 21-2.

36. Van Vuren DD, Johnson DEP. Getting started with electronic mail. Bull Med Libr Assoc 1985 Jul;73(3):267-70.

37. Dustin DC. An analysis of the QuickDOC program for management of interlibrary loans. J Interlibr Loan Inf Supply 1991;1(3):49-58.

38. Loansome Doc: a document ordering feature of Grateful Med. Bethesda, MD: National Library of Medicine, April 1991. (National Library of Medicine fact sheet).

39. National Library of Medicine Library Operations monthly report, op. cit.

40. Jackson ME. Library to library: ILL: issues and actions. Wilson Libr Bull 1991 Feb;65(6):102-5.

41. High performance computing act of 1991, Pub. L. No. 102-194, 105 Stat. 1594 (1991).

42. Braid A. Developments in facsimile and document delivery. In: Collier M, ed. Telecommunications for information management and transfer: proceedings of the first international conference held at Leicester Polytechnic, April 1987. Brookfield, VT: Gower, 1988:174-86.

43. DOCUSER file. November 1994.

44. Braid, op. cit., 174.

45. Braid A. Document delivery - the dawn of a new era. IATUL Q 1989 Dec;3(4):207-13.

46. Campbell R, Stern B. ADONIS: the publishing process moves on. Br Book News 1988 Jul;490-2.

47. Barden P. ADONIS - the British Library experience. Interlending Doc Supply 1990 Jul;18(3):88-91.

48. Stern BT, Compier HCJ. ADONIS - document delivery in the CD-ROM age. Interlending Doc Supply 1990 Jul;18(3):79-87.

49. Barden, op. cit., 89-90.

50. Stern, op. cit., 84.

51. Jackson ME. Using Ariel, RLG's document transmission system to improve document delivery in the United States. Interlending Doc Supply 1992 Apr;20(2):49-52.

52. How Romulus saves you time and money. CISTI News 1993 Dec;11(3):6.

53. Lacroix EM. SAIL: automating interlibrary loan. Bull Med Libr Assoc 1994 Apr;82(2):171-5.

54. Kennedy S. The role of commercial document delivery services in interlibrary loan. Interlending Doc Supply 1987 Jul;15(3):67-73.

55. Lenzini RT, Shaw W. UnCover and UnCover2: an article citation database and service featuring document delivery. Interlending Doc Supply 1992 Jan;20(1):12-5.

56. Use Internet to UnCover... [advertisement]. MLA News 1994 Oct;(269):22.

57. Burwell HP, Hill CN. The Burwell directory of information brokers. [10th ed.] Houston: Burwell Enterprises, 1993:v.

58. Lacroix EM. NLM Reading Room use [internal report]. December 1990.

59. Khalil M. Document delivery: a better option? Libr J 1993 Feb 1;118(2):143-7.

60. Kennedy, op. cit., 70.

61. Kilgour FG. Interlibrary loans on-line. Libr J 1979 Feb 15;104(4):460-3.

62. McGaugh DLA. The effect of DOCLINE on interlibrary loan volume and patterns among health sciences libraries in Michigan: preliminary analysis. Bull Med Libr Assoc 1990 Apr;78(2):124-30.

63. National Library of Medicine programs and services. Bethesda, MD: The Library, 1987.

64. National Library of Medicine Library Operations monthly report, op. cit.

65. National Library of Medicine programs and services, op. cit., 13.

66. National Library of Medicine Library Operations monthly report, op. cit.

67. Khalil, op. cit.,144.

68. Roche MM. ARL/RLG interlibrary loan cost study: a joint effort by the Association of Research Libraries and the Research Libraries Group. Washington, DC: Association of Research Libraries, 1993:iv.

69. Boucher V. Interlibrary loan practices handbook. Chicago: American Library Association, 1984:5,44,118.

4

Fee-Based Services

James Curtis and N.J. Wolfe

The practice of charging fees for library services has aroused much debate in the profession, especially during the past decade. In times of financial constraint, more and more libraries must wrestle with this issue. The questions surrounding service fees are complex and far-reaching, and there is considerable variation even in the definition of fee-based services. The approach to charging for services often may vary according to library type, e.g., publicly funded versus privately funded, or hospital versus academic. The scope of services for which fees are charged is quite broad and the intended clientele for these services ranges all the way from primary users to nonaffiliated individuals to corporate customers. Even the purposes underlying the charging of fees encompass widely differing motivations: to discourage use, to recoup costs, to maintain current services, to add new services and resources, or even to support the library's development program.

This chapter reviews these issues and presents a broad view of the planning and implementation process for operating certain fee-based services. Concentration will be on several of the more traditional functional areas of library service, but some attention will be devoted to a few of the newer technology-driven activities. The services to be treated include membership and access programs; photocopy, interlibrary loan and document delivery services; and less traditional programs such as media production, graphics and desktop publishing support services, and printing.

Certain other services for which fees frequently are charged will not be covered in this chapter, including specialized reference services, online search services, selective dissemination of information, and educational services. These are discussed in other volumes in this series. This division follows the traditional alignment of library departments which underlies the organization of these volumes. However, it should be noted that any given fee-based service may well cut across these boundaries. For example, there are excellent reasons to link end-user searching to automated document delivery, charging a fee for access to a locally mounted database plus a charge for copies of the documents retrieved. This approach would certainly blur the lines between access, reference, and document delivery but might provide an attractive and marketable package for a fee-based service.

There are many aspects of fee-based services that may be considered independently of the specific service setting. In addition to planning, these include business operations, legal issues, marketing of services, and evaluation.

Definitions of Fee-Based Service

What is meant by the term "fee-based service?" Are "fee-for-service" and "fee-based service" interchangeable terms? Why is the charging of fees treated as a relatively new development? After all, many libraries have long charged fees for a variety of reasons. Society libraries in nineteenth century America were largely supported by membership fees. Notable among this type of library have been the important medical society libraries such as the New York Academy of Medicine and the College of Physicians of Philadelphia. Social libraries and subscription libraries were supported by fees and are seen as the progenitors of the public library in the United States. There have been special rental collections within public libraries which charged for the circulation of best sellers or attached a fee to the use of videocassettes. Fines might be seen as a kind of fee, and nearly all public and academic libraries charge for photocopying. Libraries frequently charge each other for interlibrary loan transactions. The National Network of Libraries of Medicine (NN/LM) tied together by DOCLINE with a nationwide maximum fee for resource libraries set by the National Library of Medicine (NLM) is a prime example.

While these instances constitute fee-for-service, essential elements of true fee-based service are missing. One possible distinguishing characteristic of fee-based service is that it seeks to recoup more than the direct costs involved in the service. Josephine offers this definition as applied to the academic setting.

University library fee-based services charge a fee in addition to the direct costs incurred to obtain information for clients. This service fee may include all or part of the direct and indirect costs associated with the service. The fees may be applied to everyone regardless of their affiliation or, in some cases, fees are only charged to non-primary clientele [1].

The user of a service is viewed by several authors as central to their understanding of fee-based service. In a recent doctoral dissertation which studied the characteristics of those running fee-based services in academic libraries, Nshaiwat defines fee-based information service as "service activities made available to the public in exchange for a fee" [2] and lists qualifying services. Here the author is confining fee-based services to nonprimary clientele, which is a fairly common practice. Downing makes a similar distinction when writing about services of the New York Academy of Medicine Library.

> The term 'fee-based service' is applied narrowly to denote a service such as online searching, reference, or document delivery provided to 'fee payers' (i.e., corporate or individual *external* users who are not members of the library's defined primary clientele) for cost recovery or profit [3].

However, it appears that there is little agreement that the targeted audience determines that a service is fee-based. Restricting fee-based services to "outsiders" is not universal. Special libraries and some health sciences libraries charge back services to individuals, groups, projects, or cost centers within their parent organizations. Many libraries charge even their primary users or the user's work unit some fee for online search services. It was in fact the advent of online searching and the attempt to offset some of the costs involved with this service that opened the door for fee charging in libraries [4].

Another potential indicator of a fee-based service might be the presence of some characteristic organizational or administrative structure. Unfortunately, once again wide variability appears to be associated with such services.

> Fee-based services vary from large operations handling thousands of transactions each year, their staff supported entirely by revenue generated from clients...to small services operated as part of another library unit and expected to recover only the cost of hourly employees. In some cases, the fee-based service has no separate identity; some libraries simply have a policy to charge for document delivery or certain types of research services [5].

This definition comes very close to seeing any service for which there is a charge as a fee-based service.

For the purposes of this chapter, it is important that a clear definition of fee-based service be established. Fee-based services are a single service or a set of services, a product or products, or some combination of services and products for which a library has an established fee structure designed to recover more than direct out-of-pocket costs and which are intended for a defined user group or groups. The three essential elements of this definition are 1) set services or products; 2) fees in excess of direct costs; and 3) a clearly defined market. The fee-based service is essentially a businesslike enterprise within the library. In contrast, fee-for-service would include any service for which a library charges, including fee-based services as well as those which are not designed to recover costs.

One service which should be explicitly excluded from this definition is routine interlibrary loan. Library-to-library service for which nominal fees are charged by the lending institution fall outside this understanding of fee-based service. This is a transaction between libraries, not between libraries and users, and involves a fee which, in most cases, does not approach the true cost of the process [6]. However, if a library charges its users in excess of direct cost for interlibrary borrowing on their behalf, then this service could meet the criteria that have been established.

It should be said that there is not universal agreement that, to qualify for consideration as a fee-based service, charges must be in excess of the direct cost of providing the service. There is a school of thought which would allow any service that involves a charge to users to be accepted as a fee-based service. However, the authors do not view the simple passing on of charges incurred in providing a service, such as those paid to an online vendor or to a document delivery service, as true fee-based service. In fact, this practice should be considered as fee-for-service as distinct from fee-based service. Such practices are extremely common and seldom sufficiently organized to merit the kind of treatment outlined here. Little special planning is required to operate such services, they are generally not run like a business, and they are unlikely to be truly marketed. The use of such services benefits the vendor, who receives payment with money collected for them by the library, and the user, who receives the service at cost, but this is unlikely to increase the income of the library. Such services, in fact, cost the library if only because they fail to recover administrative and operational costs.

Though as has been stated, some would restrict fee-based services to those provided to nonprimary users or to those outside of the library's parent institution, the definition provided in this chapter does not do so. Depending on the political climate in the larger organization, the financial relationship of the library to its institution (e.g., is it expected to raise some or all of its own budget?), the willingness of the user to pay for what are perceived as value-added services, or even the strength of the desire for certain special services, the library may wish to charge even primary clientele for some services or products. In some instances these primary users are the only customer pool or target market for what the library offers. This situation may especially be the case in hospital libraries which usually only provide services to hospital-based staff and often have no external users. In any setting in which both primary users and outside clients are to be charged, it may be advisable to establish fee structures that provide for lower fees for primary users, while charging more to outside clients. Services that charge primary users in the absence of a secondary clientele or in addition to charging outside users do fall within the definition of fee-based services being used in this chapter. In fact there may be major opportunities involved in the internal market.

Free vs. Fee: Ethical and Historical Background

Philosophical arguments over charging for information have been quite sharp, especially since proponents on either side of the issue may represent widely varying institutional perspectives. There is a definite bias in favor of freedom of access to information within the library profession. This is embodied in the American Library Association's *Policy Manual* [7]. Perhaps following this lead, the Medical Library Association has adopted "A Code of Ethics for Health Sciences Librarianship" which would obligate members of the association "to promote access to health information for all" [8]. There is a strong sense within the library profession that charging fees for information services is discriminatory, especially in institutions supported by public funds [9]. However, there seems to be some variance in adherence to this value depending upon library type.

The argument against fees for library services is most fervently upheld in the public library and, to a somewhat lesser extent, by academic and health sciences libraries which receive public support, such as those in state universities and academic medical centers. The tradition of the public library as the "university of the common man" is still strongly held and abhors what it sees as inequitable barriers to access based upon ability to pay. In fact, thirty-seven states have written statutes that require public libraries to be "free" at the county or municipal level, and usually at both [10]. However, spurred on by the advent of new technologies, most especially by the availability of electronic database searching, the question of free or fee has gained increasing attention by public librarians. It is also becoming clear that fees are increasingly acceptable in the current political and economic climate. As Giacomo says in *The Fee or Free Decision*, "User fees appear to be an idea whose political time has come. They have garnered wide public support as a means for funding locally provided services, especially when considered as an option to increasing taxes" [11]. This scenario seems particularly true when the fees are attached to new services, rather than being imposed on previously free activities.

Today there are increasing numbers of fee-based services operating in public libraries. Some of the best known are targeted at businesses and offer specialized research, document delivery, and products such as patent information and market research. Notable among this type of service are FYI at the County of Los Angeles Public Library and Cleveland Research Center at the Cleveland Public Library [12]. The New York Public Library's Research Library is currently developing SIBL, a science, industry, and business library targeting the international business community in the New York City area.

Academic libraries, both public and private, also have a tradition of providing services to their faculty, staff, and students free of charge, or at least in the case of students, at no cost in addition to normal tuition and fees. Here again exceptions began to be made with the advent of computerized literature searching. Many academic libraries also participate in resource sharing agreements that attempt to eliminate or reduce interlibrary charges for materials and especially for transaction fees, thus minimizing the need to pass on costs to primary clientele for such services as interlibrary loan [13].

For some time, however, academic libraries have been responding to demands for access and services from nonprimary clientele by developing various charging mechanisms such as access or privilege cards and specialized fee-based services. These services have been on the increase since the 1960s. The first conference on Fee-Based Research in College and University Libraries was held in June 1982 [14]. This gathering spawned an Association of College and Research Libraries (ACRL) Discussion Group on Fee-Based Information Service Centers in Academic Libraries (FISCAL), which first met in 1983 [15]. At the end of 1988 the Association of Research Libraries (ARL) conducted a survey of fifty-nine of its members, all of them libraries at public universities. Seventy-nine percent responded that they had fee-based services [16]. This high percentage was in spite of the fact that many publicly funded universities have identified their mission with service to the people of their state and typically allow private citizens access to their library collections and most of their services. In many cases this access does not come without a cost, at least to some. Private university libraries have been even less reluctant to charge nonprimary users and have done so in large numbers for years, initially also for access in most cases.

Charging nonprimary clientele for simple access and borrowing privileges represents the low end of the range of operations which have been established in academic libraries. There are now major fee-based units in many university libraries offering a combination of services. Most offer, in addition to access and borrowing privileges, literature searching, current awareness service, research consultation, customized reports, and document delivery. Customers for these services include individuals, corporations, law firms, and nonprofit agencies. Among the academic libraries most visible in the field are those of the University of Michigan, Georgia Institute of Technology, Purdue University, George Washington University, Rice University, and the University of Colorado [17]. Some university and college libraries also charge fees to their primary users, but the tendency still is to heavily subsidize service to students, faculty, and staff.

Health sciences libraries, from NLM to the one-person hospital library, have shared in the tradition of free access to information, but they also have been moving increasingly into the realm of fee-for-service. In fact, health sciences libraries have probably moved further and faster in terms of instituting cost recovery schemes than many other library types, at least until recent years. There are several reasons for this earlier adoption of fees in health sciences libraries. Mention has already been made of medical society and association libraries that were supported by membership fees from their inception. The programs and services of the NLM have played an important role in the widespread adoption of fees in health sciences libraries, largely due to the fluctuations in federal funding for their support. Perhaps the three most important factors contributing to these developments were the Medical Library Assistance Act of 1965 (MLAA) and two programs which the MLAA had a hand in supporting: the Regional Medical Library (RML) Program and MEDLARS (Medical Literature Analysis and Retrieval System).

This is not the place to recount the history of these two key programs, but it is essential to recognize their importance in relation to the fee-for-service issue and the continuing movement toward fee-based services [18]. The RML Program encouraged interlibrary resource sharing by setting up regional networks of medical libraries and by providing direct subsidies for interlibrary loans. When these subsidies were removed between 1978 and 1980, most health sciences libraries began charging each other for interlibrary lending, and many started passing these costs for borrowing along to their users. Similarly the expansion of access to MEDLINE was supported by the MLAA, and by 1973 the costs of this program too began to be passed on to the MEDLINE search centers which, in turn, established fees for their users.

The direct costs of technology made recovering some of the costs necessary. During the second half of the 1970s, libraries began charging fees for such services as computer searching and photocopying. By 1979, income from services had become important enough to be documented in the the the Association of Academic Health Sciences Library Directors (AAHSLD) statistics. Over 3% of the average library's revenues were from "fee-for-service" [19].

While this was the picture in academic health sciences libraries, the situation was slightly different in most hospital library settings. Naturally these same events of the 1960s and 70s had their effect on them, but they did not necessarily respond in the same way. While virtually all academic health sciences libraries began passing along costs for online literature searching to their users, and some instituted charges for interlibrary borrowing, these practices were less common among hospital libraries. In Bloomquist's *Library Practice in Hospitals: A Basic Guide,* published in 1972, there is no mention of charges to users even in the chapters on interlibrary loan and MEDLARS [20]. By 1983, when *Hospital Library Management* was published, it is stated that "at present, most hospital libraries do not charge for interlibrary loan service. Increases in the volume of loans and in costs associated with both borrowing and lending may require, however, that charging for this service be considered" [21]. In discussing online searching, Messerle declares that "many libraries choose to incorporate these costs into the library budget and provide free online searches as part of the overall reference function." She goes on to say that other systems do exist, including cost recovery, adding a profit factor, and charging either individual users or charging back to departments [22]. Still the impression is left that charging fees for these services was relatively uncommon in hospitals.

Looking at the fourth edition of the *Handbook of Medical Library Practice,* which appeared between 1982 and 1988, one will find very little reference to charging fees for service and no mention of true fee-based service of the type then becoming more common in academic libraries. Brief mention is made of charging nonprimary users for access. Support for this practice seems lukewarm, however, as it is noted that the procedure of establishing fees for use of the collection by outside users is occasionally resented [23]. Mention is made of the possibility of full cost recovery for interlibrary loan and document delivery to nonprimary users and of a potential shift from full subsidy to partial cost recovery for primary users [24]. The chapter on reference services discusses fees only in the context of charging for the cost of online literature searches and is rather equivocal on the advisability and fairness of doing so [25]. In the section on searching and search techniques the subject of charging is treated with great caution, leaving the impression that it should be avoided if at all possible [26]. Whatever the philosophical misgivings about charging for services, a study that was conducted in 1978 of 708 U.S. and Canadian institutions using the NLM's search services showed that 53% of the respondents charged for online searches. This percentage varied, based on library type, with 91% of educational institution libraries charging while only 34% of hospital library respondents charged [27].

Despite a reluctance to charge that seems apparent among health sciences librarians, there is evidence that change has been in the wind for several years. *Cost Analysis, Cost Recovery, Marketing, and Fee-based Services: A Guide for the Health Sciences Librarian,* edited by Wood, appeared in 1985 and remains an excellent primer on fee-based reference services, particularly in the chapters that deal with principles rather than those that describe specific programs. Much of this work is devoted to true cost recovery programs that seek to offset both direct and indirect costs rather than simply to pass on out-of-pocket charges incurred in providing services. Several fee-based operations that offer services to nonprimary users are also described or mentioned, most notably those at the Louis Calder Memorial Library at the University of Miami, the Biomedical Information Service of the University of Minnesota's Bio-Medical Library, and the fee-for-service component of the Cleveland Health Sciences Library [28].

Additional evidence of the expanding attention to fee-based services among health sciences librarians came with the formation of a fee-based special interest group within the Public Services Section of the Medical Library Association. This group held its first informal gathering during the 1987 Annual Meeting. While little has been written to date describing the extent of fee-based service provision in hospital libraries, extensive membership by hospital librarians in this new group may indicate a growing interest.

Entrepreneurship and Intrapreneurship

A major factor in the success of any fee-based service is the existence of the entrepreneurial spirit. Entrepreneurs are individuals who conceive a venture, define and organize it, arrange its financing, and assume the risk that is associated with the undertaking. Risk is a significant consideration when launching an entrepreneurial service or business, and while risk does carry the chance of failure, it also implies the possibility of substantial success.

The business literature is filled with references to entrepreneurship in the corporate arena. Spirited individuals have left their comfortable positions to go off on their own and develop new companies to meet the changing needs of the public. Because of these success stories, many established corporations have encouraged and supported entrepreneurial activities within their traditional operations to improve their market share and to address newly emerging needs. This incorporation of entrepreneurship within existing organizations is called intrapreneurship and is a potentially useful model for libraries.

Unfortunately, risk taking is somewhat contrary to the typical behavior of most librarians and library management. Libraries wanting to take advantage of intrapreneurial activities will need to overcome the characteristic low-risk approach to managerial style. According to Drucker, too much risk avoidance is counterproductive. "The attempt to eliminate risks, even the attempt to minimize them, can only make them irrational and unbearable. It can only result in the greatest risk of all: rigidity" [29].

Entrepreneurial managers must have this risk taking attitude, coupled with ideas. The term "change agent" has many times been used to describe this type of individual. The manager who promotes change serves as a role model for other library staff who become involved in the fee-based endeavors of a library. Staff should be empowered and given the necessary resources to accomplish the transformation in services that will be offered to library users. Managers of fee-based services must inspire and nurture their staffs to insure that they reach their full potential. Vision, flexibility, and creativity are necessary strengths in a manager charged with the task of developing a fee-based service. Such innovative approaches to librarianship may pave the way for the services of the twenty-first century, including those based on fees.

Teamwork is an essential requirement for the pursuit of entrepreneurial goals. The idea of participatory management is not new, but it is of increased importance in nurturing fee-based services. Management must encourage the entrepreneurial effort to be built with a cohesive and committed team effort. Only in a climate of trust and shared responsibility will fee-based services ever have any hope of success. Existing library staff will in most cases be reluctant to change unless they are closely involved in research, development, and the change process. Cargill and Webb state that "developing effective teams will facilitate organizational change" and will be especially useful in transitional libraries [30].

Types of Fee-Based Services

The scope of this chapter is restricted to dealing with only a few types of fee-based services. These are the services that fall within the sphere of access and delivery in health sciences libraries. Specifically, this chapter deals with membership or access programs, with photocopy and document delivery services, including some aspects of interlibrary borrowing, and with some special library services such as media or graphics production and printing of computer output. The common thread is that each of these services relates either to using the collections or obtaining a "product" from the library.

While it would be possible to provide a long list of services and products for which libraries currently charge, this has been done and would also involve listing many which are beyond the scope of this chapter [31]. For a comprehensive international listing of fee-based services, their products, and research areas, *The FISCAL Directory of Fee-Based Research and Document Supply Services* is an invaluable and extremely informative resource with profiles of hundreds of services [32].

Most fee-based operations offer a combination of specific services and products. Membership or access programs for nonprimary users could be restricted to admission to the library and use of collections, but they commonly involve the use of other library systems and services as well. In particular, access programs often include the use of reference services, research consultation, and online search services. The combination of access and document delivery does make a logical set of services, but it may lack that higher level of professional intervention which distinguishes good public service in health sciences libraries.

Membership and Access Programs

Membership or access programs are almost always designed to extend certain library privileges to nonprimary users. At a minimum, they include allowing unaffiliated users into the library and the on-site use of the library's collections. They may include limited or full circulation privileges. The use of some or all of the library's systems, equipment, and services may also be part of the package. Generally, access alone is provided for a fixed fee, with other privileges being charged for incrementally and at a combination of fixed and variable rates. Usually the membership or access program user will pay for these other library services at a higher rate than that paid by primary users.

Membership programs are sometimes designed to contribute to the library's development or public relations efforts [33]. Access to collections and services can be given as a benefit for those contributing to the library's fund-raising programs. Contributors or members of the friends of the library group might be charged reduced rates for library services. The access program might contribute to the public relations efforts of the library by providing the means for businesses and individuals to take advantage of the information and services the library has to offer. Most likely there will be some impact on the access service fee structure if development or outreach is part of its goal. In other words, "membership has its privileges."

Access programs are often seen as possible only in a private institution. It is true that the optimum conditions for operating such programs are more likely to be present in a private setting, where control over who even gets into the building can be fairly tight. In institutions that are publicly funded it may not be possible or wise to restrict entry. This does not mean that once inside all services are available to the unaffiliated user. It may be possible to charge a fee for borrowing privileges. Access to other services such as mediated searching and photocopy may cost more for the unaffiliated user. Business users and commercial information brokers may also be charged at higher rates than the private citizen. Whether private or public, it would be prudent to consult with the legal staff of one's institution at an early stage in planning for charging for any service to be certain that the proposed policies will stand up if challenged.

A broad view of access should also include electronic access. Library catalogs and locally mounted databases can often be freely accessed on a dial-in basis or over the Internet. Typically there is no charge for this and little means of controlling who gets access. This does not have to be the case, however, and there are opportunities for creation of fee-based electronic access programs. All that is needed is that remote users be required to obtain passwords in order to connect to library systems and that a fee be charged for this access. At first thought, this may seem overly restrictive. However, when taken to the next step, control of access, identification of users, and charging of fees seems eminently logical. That next step is to attach a delivery order system to the catalog or database. This cannot be done unless individual users can be identified to the system.

Photocopy, Document Delivery, and Interlibrary Loan

Mediated photocopy, document delivery, and interlibrary borrowing form a functionally connected cluster of services related to production and distribution of information products. All deal with obtaining library materials for users, some in the form of photocopies and some in the form of actual books or journals. The primary differences among these services are the sources from which the materials originate and the means by which they are obtained and delivered. Interestingly enough, these differences all exist behind the scenes, out of sight to library users. This is one reason why it is desirable to integrate these services so that the user can ask for an item and receive it without necessarily having to negotiate the rules governing what may appear to them as an arcane set of overlapping services.

At a minimum, photocopy services perform the actual copying of materials from the library's collections and turn them over to the user. In this case the materials are located, retrieved, and taken to the service by the user who later picks up the finished copies. From this base the service may add several features. It could receive orders by various written or electronic means, pull the materials, copy them, and deliver them back to the user. The delivery mechanism might be part of the photocopy service or of a linked document delivery service.

A document delivery service will require a photocopying component to produce copies of materials from the library's collections, but it is likely to offer some other services as well. It may deliver books. It may obtain materials in either photocopy or the original from other nearby, possibly affiliated libraries such as branch or departmental libraries. The delivery service might go outside of the home library and the institution to obtain materials from other libraries through interlibrary borrowing or from commercial document suppliers. A complete document delivery service receives requests from users for specific items, identifies a source for the items, obtains them by various means, and delivers them to the user by one of a number of methods which they have selected.

A delivery service might be available to the library's primary users, to nonprimary users, or to anyone who is able to pay the fees. Primary library users are more likely to accept being charged for document delivery when it is an additional service beyond what are considered to be standard library functions previously provided free of charge. When delivery services go beyond provision of materials from their own collections to their own base user group, they enter increasingly problematic legal territory, some of it not well-charted. The complications are associated with interlibrary loan codes, copyright laws, tax codes, and laws governing competition with the private sector. Professional legal help will be needed if this broad type of service is contemplated.

Electronic access and delivery services make an increasingly appealing package for the fee-based service operator and the user alike. Loansome Doc, NLM's system to allow electronic access by users through Grateful Med to their primary libraries, and through them to the DOCLINE network, could serve as a key element in a fee-based service for any size library. Several nationwide commercial and not-for-profit services currently exist. Examples of these are UnCover, OCLC's FirstSearch, and the Research Libraries Group (RLG)'s CitaDel. More such services are on the horizon. Similar types of service are by no means beyond the capability of many academic medical centers. Even for the smaller library, the ability to display holdings in various CD-ROM databases has brought the possibility of a customized order system one step closer. Many online catalog systems also incorporate a request capability into their OPACs. These new system features could easily be incorporated into a fee-based document delivery service, thus making it possible for virtually any library to go into business.

Other Services

There are several less conventional services that have fee-based potential in health sciences libraries. These are linked to the capabilities of the microcomputer. Many libraries have long had media or learning resources services. During the last ten years these have changed from collections of audiovisuals into microcomputer centers. Along with the increased potential for interactive learning that has come with this evolution, there is also the opportunity to develop new fee-based services. Microcomputers in the library are often used for word processing, spreadsheet applications, bibliographic formatting, and desktop publishing, as well as for computer-assisted instruction. Each of these applications at least potentially requires expertise that might be provided by a paid consultant. High-quality printing may provide another niche with the potential for charging a fee. Data often needs to be represented graphically, printed components of poster session presentations need to be produced, illustrations and other materials need to be scanned, and electronic formats need to be converted. Custom-printed products from OPACs, CD-ROM databases, and other bibliographic and nonbibliographic sources could be done for a charge. The enterprising librarian may take advantage of these needs to build a service that provides assistance or products to its users for a fee.

Planning for Fee-Based Services

Adequate initial planning for fee-based services is an important first step toward success. A thorough job done at this stage can help the library avoid many problems during implementation of a new service. Planning has several aspects. These include determination of the appropriate financial model for the service, setting goals for the service, performing an internal assessment, conducting market research, and defining policy issues.

Alternative Financial Models

Library services may be grouped according to their source of financial support into four basic categories: subsidized services, partially subsidized services, cost recovery services, and entrepreneurial services. These categories relate to the definition of fee-based service as outlined earlier in this chapter. Examples of fully subsidized services usually include most of those traditionally provided by libraries, such as access to the building and collections, reference desk services, circulation services, the catalog, and core collections. If interlibrary borrowing is done without a charge to the user, it also falls into the fully subsidized category. These services are completely supported by the library's base resources, and they generate virtually no offsetting income.

Partially subsidized services are those earlier defined as fee-for-service. These services are established using base resources. There is a cost to the user for these services, but the charge only equals out-of-pocket expenses, such as vendor charges for online searching, or the charge may be for all direct costs and some indirect costs. Examples of partially subsidized services might include most mediated search services or workshops for primary users. In most cases interlibrary lending is a subsidized service since full costs are not recovered [34].

The final two financial models comprise those which the authors consider to be fee-based service. The first is cost recovery services which also may originate with support from the library's base budget, but which must become fully supported by user fees and require no continuing subsidy from the base budget resources. These might include photocopy services, full-cost interlibrary lending and borrowing, specialized research services and products, and document delivery services.

The final category of services is entrepreneurial. These are services that are established using resources outside of the library's budget base. The funding might derive from grant support or from special onetime start-up support given by a library's parent institution, such as the university or the hospital, or from some special fund-raising effort. Once started, the entrepreneurial program is expected to support itself without subsidy and perhaps even return some revenue in excess of costs to the library to reinvest in the service or to be used elsewhere. Any kind of service might be founded on this basis, but the more common ones are specialized reference and consultation services and electronic and other quick turn-around document delivery services.

Services may migrate or mature from one category into another. Most services grow out of an extension of traditional library services to new groups of users or an evolution into more highly specialized or individualized services. These often start out as fully or partially subsidized. For example, membership or access programs clearly depend on the preexisting core resource of the library and its collections. Document delivery services may well evolve from a base in mediated photocopy services and interlibrary loan. Some of these services may progress all the way into profit-making services, bringing in more than the direct and indirect costs combined. Making or appearing to make a profit can be problematic for libraries. If not handled properly this could jeopardize whatever tax exempt status the library might enjoy. Making a profit may not even be allowable, particularly in public institutions. These issues will be further discussed later in this chapter.

It is extremely useful at an early stage in the planning of any new service to determine the intended category of financial support as outlined in these models. This will help to inform the internal assessment and to answer such questions as which existing services show potential for becoming fee-based and how start-up funding will be obtained. Establishing the goal during initial planning of becoming at least a cost recovery operation will help to guide many of the practical decisions that must be made along the way.

Setting Goals

Setting clear goals for a new service is a very important part of the planning phase. A fee-based service is likely to have two sets of goals, one being financial, the other expressed in terms of services to be provided [35]. The model outlined previously helps simplify the task of setting financial goals. Since fee-based services have here been defined as quite literally services based upon or financed by fees, this type of service should strive to achieve cost recovery status. Therefore the financial goal of a fee-based service might be, "To provide X services to Y users for fees which will cover all costs to the library, both direct and indirect, without detriment to existing library services."

Some services which charge fees and may even be called fee-based will not realistically be able to recover all costs. Access services for nonprimary users are the major example. The resource that makes access and membership services possible is the entire library. Certainly this cost is too great to even contemplate recovering. This complicates both the setting of goals for access service and the process of setting fees. The topic of price-setting is closely related to the financial goal of a service and will be addressed elsewhere in full; it may be said at this point that given a goal of recovering all direct and indirect costs for provision of a service, the manager has a fairly good chance of figuring out what to charge. Since it is impossible in the case of access services to cover all the costs that might be associated with the service, the goal can at best be to recover direct costs of the new program plus some additional factor, an arrangement sometimes called cost-plus.

The specification of service goals comprises the other component of goal setting for fee-based services and is probably an area where the librarian will feel more at ease. This sense of comfort could prove dangerous if it leads to inadequate attention to this important phase of planning. This is the point at which one must state what will be done and for whom in terms that can be understood by all. Once again clarity at this point will help to guide actual policy and procedure development as the service is later designed in detail. Even at this early stage of planning for a fee-based service, it is advisable to be as explicit as possible about what will be included. For instance, in an access program will all services of the library be available to clients once a single fee has been paid? Will some services be excluded? Will there be additional fees for certain services? Should services for primary clientele remain unchanged and undisturbed by addition of the fee-based service?

Delivery services run a particularly high risk of being disruptive of normal library operations. For instance, if a new service is started using existing staff, the priorities for handling orders originating from different sources may be upset. Increased competition for items in the collection and for photocopy resources may be created. The urgency associated with the fee-based service requests may threaten established orderly procedures. If this situation is to be avoided, a clear intention to leave existing services unaffected should be expressed in the goal statement. It is important that service goals be clear not only to those outside of the library, including the potential customers for services, but also to the library staff who may have apprehensions about the advent of new and different services and for institutional administrators who may need to approve the library's plans.

Service goals will not be complete until the intended users for a fee-based service have been identified. This is an important first step in targeting the market for a new operation. It is possible with this part of the goal-setting process, as well as in service definition, that the targeted users and intended service will need to be modified based upon what is learned during later stages of planning and implementation activities. It is good to be flexible, but advisable to begin with fairly concrete objectives in mind. The major decision related to users of a fee-based service is to determine if the service is for primary users, nonprimary users, or for nonusers. All three may be the intended audience, but once again this decision will have important ramifications in setting up and running the service. The greatest effort both in terms of early market research and in later marketing will be required if the target is individuals or groups who have not previously been users of the library's services.

Internal Assessment

It is absolutely necessary at an early stage of planning for a fee-based service to take a careful look at the library and its parent institution to determine in as objective a manner as possible the relevant strengths and weaknesses of the organization [36]. One of the most basic problems that must be acknowledged is that the library is not fundamentally a business organization; it probably has not been set up to respond to customers in a businesslike fashion, to manage its affairs in businesslike ways, nor to pay attention to the bottom line. Regardless of how one feels about the fee or free debate, it must be admitted that libraries are, in origin, service organizations, not businesses. They deal in information and attempt to help their users by acquiring, organizing, and providing access, placing a minimum of barriers between the users and the information they need. The mission of the library and the parent institution should be examined to determine if the creation of a fee-based service might be seen to conflict with overall goals. Should it appear that there will be problems in this regard, a strategy for responding to a perceived conflict should be developed.

As part of the internal assessment, planners should be clear about the purpose for starting a fee-based service. The purpose may appear to be simple: to produce income. However, bringing in income may be a goal of creating the fee-based service or a partial result of having the service, but it may not be the purpose. As stated in the introduction to this chapter, the purpose could be to respond to external demand for service, or to exercise limits and controls on access, or to reach out to the community as part of a development strategy. Each of these purposes could result in very different service and promotion strategies.

Service planners must be very familiar with the library's collections, staff, equipment, physical plant, and with existing library services and how they are being supported. These are the potential raw materials of a fee-based service and where one may be able to discover competitive advantages that distinguish a given library from the competition. It is also in this phase of self-examination that the potential impact of a new fee-based service on existing services may begin to emerge. The intent in this process is to define strengths and weaknesses. Factors that might contribute to, or detract from, a fee-based service could include special collection strengths, location, accessibility, resident expertise, adequate machine base (e.g., photocopiers, computer workstations), and space to give the service a home.

Start-up resources should be identified during the internal assessment. One of the biggest mistakes that can be made in starting a business is to be undercapitalized. This also applies to starting a fee-based service in a library. There are likely to be extra start-up expenses that will not necessarily be recurring but must be covered initially. A sufficient income stream to allow the service to reach a goal of cost recovery will not be achieved for some time. How far is the library (or some other funding source) willing to go in subsidizing a new fee-based service? How much will it cost and for how long? Which of its resources other than budget is the library willing to extend, and under what circumstances? Can the service expect to use existing space, staff, and equipment? Will the service itself be charged for doing so? Again, the question of the relationship between existing services and new services must be carefully examined.

Libraries follow all sorts of procedures and have many policies that are tangential to the actual delivery of access and information services to users. These are the business, financial, and accounting procedures followed by the library and by its parent institution. One must not omit an examination of these policies and procedures during the internal assessment. Whether a given library exists within a hospital, an academic medical center, or even in a corporation, there are rules and regulations over which the operators of a fee-based service will have little or no control. These can present substantial obstacles to running a service that wants to encourage use and maximize efficiency. They run the gamut from work rules, to billing policies, to where revenues must end up (often in a general fund and not under the library's control). Frequently, those planning new services are insufficiently aware of these policies and procedures because they have typically not been closely involved with them until they embark on the implementation of a fee-based service. Involvement of the library's and the parent institution's business managers in the assessment and design stages is very important in creating successful fee-based services.

Market Research

There are entire courses in business schools and volumes of literature on doing market research [37]. It would be neither possible nor desirable to repeat or even summarize this material in the current chapter. There are several useful works describing market research in the library setting. Among these are *Making Money: Fees for Library Services* by Warner [38], and the chapter by Lemkau, Burrows, and La Rocco entitled "Marketing Library Services Outside the Medical Center" in Wood's guide [39].

Any discussion of marketing or market research must begin in one place: with the user. Market research is a user-centered activity, not, at least initially, a product-centered activity. Its object is to find out as much as possible about the potential users of services, what it is that they want that the library might provide, and what it would be worth to the user to obtain these services. To do this, one must start by identifying subsets of actual or potential users. It is important to recognize that not all users are alike. Of particular potential are those who might be identified as having a high interest in certain of the library's services and the means to pay for them. These users will usually be some group outside of the primary users of the library, but not always. Often the focus of research will be businesses, law firms, group medical practices, or various agencies or associations. It is also wise to begin with some known group of users with whose current needs the library has some familiarity.

Very often a library will decide what services it wants to market and go out and promote them, without much success. A principal reason for this failure may well be that the staff has acted on the assumption that it knows what users want and has guessed at what they are willing to pay. Obviously the library faces certain practical limits in regard to the services it can perform, but to decide what to offer, how it will set up its operations, and how the services will be promoted, all without adequate information about targeted users, is to stand the process on its head. Services and products must be tailored to client needs and shown to be distinct from, and superior to, competing products and services. The library must present itself as a responsive agency guided by the needs of its clients. To do or become these things, libraries need information about the clients and the competition. Libraries have usually designed their services and operations to serve a mass audience. They strive to routinize everything, to produce consistent products and services for all users, and to follow the maxim "the greatest good to the greatest number." To realize success with a fee-based service, this attitude must be changed.

The actual process of market research may involve several steps. Some can be done more or less independently; others will involve the users directly. A first step might be an assessment of environmental trends and conditions. This assessment requires an examination of the macrocosm in which the service will operate. Typical questions that might be investigated are what topics are "hot" at the moment and what kinds of information relate to these topics; who, in general, are the major consumers of information in an area; what new developments in information technology are expected over the next five years; are any major demographic shifts in the environment expected; and what competing and complementary sources of information are available in the area. This background work should also involve reviewing the literature of fee-based services, examining the annual reports of potential customers, and contacting libraries that offer these services and may be willing to share experiences.

Once the big picture has been pieced together it may be possible to develop some projections and to formulate fairly focused questions that may be pursued by seeking actual user input. Enough should have been learned through the goal-setting process, the internal assessment, and the examination of the environment to postulate the likely services and users for a new enterprise. At this point, the hypotheses will need to be tested. There are many specific techniques and methods for obtaining information about users and their reactions to proposed library services. Most of these information-gathering techniques involve asking the user directly, either through surveys or the use of focus groups.

Surveys may attempt to poll entire populations of users, or they may follow a sampling technique. They may be conducted in person, by phone, by fax, or through mailings. Some are even being conducted electronically. Whatever the method, the survey should be designed to learn about specific user or group characteristics and needs. They should also try to determine the best means for reaching the users with promotional materials and what types of appeals are most likely to succeed with them. If plans are far enough along, it may be desirable to try to gather reactions to fairly specific service proposals. Also useful, if it can be obtained, is some information on what fees the users might be willing to pay. However, trying to get this kind of information by simply asking may provide unreliable results. It may be possible to consult with experts on conducting surveys in one's institution.

Survey design is something of an art, and the novice should use whatever support resources are available [40].

Another technique for obtaining information about users is the focus group. Conducting a successful focus group is not a simple matter and may require even more expert help than designing a good survey would. One advantage of this method is that the more open format and opportunity for direct interaction may help to generate ideas and suggest ways to modify plans. It is less likely to occur as a result of a survey in which the answers to predetermined questions are sought. In fact, one approach is to use both focus group and survey techniques with the results of the former helping in the design of the latter [41].

A final technique which is part market research and part early implementation is the pilot study. Used frequently in manufacturing and product development, the pilot study might be considered a kind of prototyping. In a pilot study, a service is set up and offered under controlled conditions to validate assumptions and learn more about user acceptance before too much has been risked. While it is important to build in an evaluative process in operational services, this is absolutely essential in conducting a pilot test. Good evaluation requires that some fairly specific questions be posed and benchmarks established to determine whether the pilot has been a success or not. These goals may be expressed in terms of units of work, numbers of customers, income, processing time, user satisfaction, quality of output, or some other measures. Setting a time limit for the pilot test will also be necessary. When all this has been done, the service will reach a "go/no-go" decision point. Modification of the service may be necessary, then maybe more testing or back to the drawing board.

Policies

Having set goals, conducted an internal assessment, and completed market research, the fee-based service planner is prepared to take the first steps toward actual implementation of the service. All of the information that has been gathered will now be applied as policies for the service are developed. These policies will define the service and will help to provide a structure for its operations. Issues identified during earlier stages of planning will need to be resolved as policies are set. The issues and policies covered here address three aspects of fee-based service planning: the services that will be offered, the users of the services, and the charges for the services. Because each of these aspects is intertwined with the others, it is difficult to discuss any one in isolation. Such issues as copyright, confidentiality, and competition with the private sector are addressed in the Legal Issues section of this chapter.

Services

One of the most difficult problems with the creation of a fee-based service in a library is that the new must coexist with the old. The fee-based service is not being created and will not function in a vacuum. Ongoing library operations must not be ignored, and they may be affected by the introduction of a service which is set up to accomplish newly identified goals. This is one of the reasons that it is important to confirm that the fee-based service does not conflict with the mission of the library early on in the planning stage. Even though this may have been done, it can be difficult to set up a new operation that takes into consideration those services the library has long provided and still presents the picture of a logical whole to staff and users.

Access to the collections is a prime example of the potentially complicated multiplicity of services which may grow up in a library. Basic library services will almost certainly include circulation of items to walk-in primary users, self-service photocopying, and obtaining materials from other libraries through interlibrary borrowing. Some of these services may be free to all or have a fee attached to them which applies to some users or to everyone. A fee-based access service may include some charge for all of these services. Certain costs, like access to the collection and circulation of materials, will probably be covered by a set membership fee; other costs may be variable and be charged at a different rate than for primary users. The relationship of document delivery to interlibrary loan can also complicate matters. Might users now end up paying for delivered materials coming from their library's collections, but getting loans from another library for free because interlibrary borrowing has always been subsidized? The problem is that services tend to grow up incrementally and may not comprise the kind of rational whole that one would create if starting from scratch. Unfortunately the complex of services offered by the library may become hard for staff to understand and explain, and it may present a totally obtuse picture to users.

To avoid this, all of the library's services must be considered whenever a new service, particularly a fee-based service, is added. It is not good to confuse either the new customers one hopes to attract or an existing user base. It will be necessary to state clearly which services are free and which are fee-based and to be able to justify these policies. The services for which there is a charge will probably be new or enhanced ones, especially if both primary and nonprimary users are targeted. It is politically difficult to impose new charges on old services for primary users. If the intended users of the fee-based service are groups who have not previously been using the library, then imposing a charge on preexisting services does not present the same problems. An example of this would be the creation of a membership or access program for businesses, practice groups, or law firms who may have had no access or only limited access before the introduction of the fee-based service.

A new document delivery service will need to respond to many policy issues. The first of these is will the service be for photocopies of articles only or for books as well? Delivering photocopies is relatively easier; the documents flow one way. Books, on the other hand, must be returned. Another question to resolve is what will be the sources for the documents delivered? Will they all come from the library's own collections, from other nearby collections such as other campus libraries or consortium members, from other libraries through interlibrary borrowing, or from commercial document suppliers? As the sources spread out, the legal, financial, and service delivery challenges increase. Document delivery has great potential for complication, since it can overlay existing interlibrary loan services.

A further set of questions that must be resolved at the policy-setting stage relates to method of delivery, which may range from pickup service to personal delivery by courier. The use of the mails may be acceptable if orders are not urgent. Express mail services are also available. Fax delivery will no doubt be a popular option. Electronic delivery of online search results and special reports is widely done today, and electronic delivery of full-text literature is becoming more and more common. Turnaround time and guarantees regarding delivery of products must also be addressed as part of policy-setting. The close link between speed and method of delivery should be obvious, and speed will be one of the chief selling points for a fee-based delivery service.

Fees will probably vary according to the delivery mechanism applied to a given order, but it is reasonable to assume that a lower fee will be charged for items picked up at the library by the user than for those personally delivered to an office. Two variables are at work here: labor costs and speed. In some cases, labor costs increase as a function of speed, but in others this is not the case. Providing a range of delivery options and prices will make good sense from the marketing perspective but will complicate operations, record keeping, and billing. The planner must take all of this into consideration when setting policies to make them sensible, attractive, and a help to operations rather than a hindrance.

At the same time that delivery options are being considered it may be convenient to make decisions related to the means by which requests will be received. A range of possibilities may be offered. Requests may be personally delivered, mailed, phoned in, faxed, or sent electronically. The goal of the service should again be responsiveness, so taking requests by any of a variety of means at the choice of the user makes good business sense. However, the need for accountability for service, satisfaction of legal requirements, and tracking financial responsibility for obligations assumed may make some of the electronic means a bit problematical.

A further factor for consideration when setting service policy is the position of the new service vis-à-vis the competition. Here again market research is translated into practical terms. The fee-based service should attempt to fill some niche which has been discovered in the local market for information access and delivery. To find that niche, data about potential customers, the library, and the competition have been obtained. The service which results should be built on the user's needs, library strengths, and the competition's weaknesses. The policies which implement it should be designed to maximize the marketability of a service through flexibility and responsiveness.

Users

Much of the policy-setting for new fee-based services will revolve around the intended users of the service. As observed in the discussion about which services should be provided, it is impossible to answer that question without reference to who will be the users of the services. Perhaps the central issue here is whether the service will be intended for the library's primary users, some other group, or for both. Many fee-based services are aimed at nonprimary users. Access and membership programs only make sense as services for those who would not or could not otherwise use the library. Other types of fee-based services that are covered in this chapter, such as photocopy, document delivery, and microcomputer-related services, might be used by primary as well as outside users.

There are several issues that relate to this decision. One of these is essentially a political one: does the library wish to appear to offer a higher level of service to nonprimary users than to its existing user base? Probably not, but at the same time if the fee-based service had to offer all of its services to primary users free of charge, it would be forced to raise fees for other users and might price itself out of competitiveness. If the goal of the service is full cost recovery, as is likely, then even primary users will need to pay. The question then becomes, do they pay less than others? Should the minimum charge, even for primary users, be set at the cost recovery level, or should one set of customers subsidize another?

Decisions about the intended users for a fee-based service are likely to depend on the answer to a fundamental question: who has money and is willing to pay for the services offered? Some answers to this question should have been found during the market research phase of planning. User segments which fit the profile may have been identified among primary users, nonprimary users, and nonusers. In the academic or hospital library setting, those having funds and willing to pay for special services might include recipients of grant support or earners of significant incomes from clinical sources. Outside the institution, businesses involved in research and development, especially in biomedical fields, are good potential customers. One group of possible users may prove controversial, perhaps more so in the hospital environment than in the academic medical center library. Lawyers frequently want access to medical information and are usually willing to pay for it. However, some physician users may resent a lawyer for a plaintiff in a malpractice suit having access to the medical library. At the same time, the doctor would probably want a lawyer who defends in such cases to have access to all the information and help available. Service policies should not attempt to discriminate based on the purposes for which clients want information. Any exclusions from access to a fee-based service would have to be legally and ethically defensible. Policies may be set up to encourage or discourage certain groups, but when operating a business new legal realms are entered and some control may be forfeited.

Current technology makes it possible for the library to have users whom it never sees. These remote users have the ability to access library catalogs and other databases electronically from their homes, offices, and laboratories. If the library makes electronic ordering a feature of its fee-based service, these users could become customers without ever having to enter the library. When setting up policies for the service, this should be kept in mind. Does it make sense to allow users to find and order materials electronically but not be able to apply for privileges or pay for them without coming to the library? To take full advantage of this group of potential users, policies should be designed to allow for those who wish to conduct their business at a distance.

Setting Prices

Finally, the bottom line: what should be charged for the library's services? Many of the factors that will contribute to this decision have already been pointed out. A service is likely to charge a range of fees, some fixed, some variable. Whether a charge is fixed or variable and exactly how much it is may depend on the specific service being rendered, how it is being performed, and who the user is. Access and membership programs are likely to have a mixture of fixed and variable fees. Photocopy and document delivery services can have variable or per page fees, but might also have a minimum fixed fee per transaction. Other services such as media or graphics production may have a per job charge. Whatever the particular arrangement, once again the object of charging in a fee-based service is the same, to recover costs.

Determining costs and setting prices for services are key elements contributing to the success or failure of an operation. Perhaps more than any other factor this requires that the librarian adopt a businesslike attitude. Arbitrary price-setting and overly complex fee structures should be avoided. Attention should be paid to what the competition is charging, but this cannot be the most important consideration in setting fees.

There are two kinds of costs involved in providing library services: direct costs and indirect costs. Direct costs are those specifically identified with an activity and include labor and materials and supplies, with labor accounting for the bulk of the costs. One could compute the labor needed to perform every job on each occasion and come up with quite exact costs, which would vary from job to job. This method is known as job costing; while accurate, it may not be practical for many operations. Instead one should attempt to determine standard labor costs involved in providing a given service. These should remain fairly constant over the course of many jobs. In other words, labor costs for a service should average out over time. One way to do this is to compute the average unit of time spent by each of various staff members on a sample of jobs in fractions of hours and multiply their total hourly compensation by this amount. This method is known as process costing. Either method should provide similar results if the staffing level is appropriate. Material and supply costs may also be figured on a per job basis or an average may be determined. The per unit average or per hour average methods are preferable [42].

Indirect costs present the greatest problem because by definition they are not entirely assignable to the fee-based service. These are costs such as certain collection and collection maintenance costs, light, heat, and other physical plant expenses, equipment shared with other services, and any administrative costs which cannot be directly assigned. One approach is to establish some formula that distributes indirect costs across all library services, attaching them to each separate service in proportion to its share of the total services provided by the library. There are various methods for doing this, but one example is to assign indirect costs according to the proportion of staff members in a given service to the total library staff. Equipment costs may comprise a special category of cost assignable to the service or may be part of the indirect cost. The choice would depend on whether the equipment was purchased for the fee-based service and is used exclusively by it, or is an item shared with other library services.

The initial setting of prices may involve a certain amount of guesswork no matter how much cost and customer analysis has gone into the decision making. It may be that actual costs will vary from estimates. Users may prove unwilling to pay the prices, or the volume of business may not be what was predicted. Whatever happens, it is very important to monitor costs and revenues closely and be prepared to make adjustments as they are needed. It is also important, however, to recognize that circumstances during the start-up phase of the service will differ from those experienced in a more mature operation. One does not want to start making too many adjustments too soon. If the initial research and planning have been done well, it is best to trust their results for a while. One cannot expect that cost recovery status will be achieved overnight, and therefore it is imperative that a new fee-based service have adequate start-up funding.

Operating Fee-Based Services

Organization and Administration

The organization and administration of fee-based services follow no single model. These services vary from large nearly autonomous operations to virtual sidelines within library departments that have other major responsibilities. The manner in which any particular service will be organized and administered will depend on a number of factors including the overall size of the library, the type of services being offered, the expected volume, the goals of the service, and the method and amount of financing available to support the start-up of the service.

The major decision to be made with regard to organization of a fee-based service hinges on its relationship to other library departments, or to the library itself in the case of smaller libraries. Will the fee-based service comprise a separate department, or will it be added onto an existing department? If it is to be added on, to which department? What will be the effect of one arrangement versus another? Certain types of service are more easily treated as add-on services than others. Access programs that involve no or very few additional services may be subsumed under the library unit responsible for administering library privileges with fairly modest repercussions. Promotion of the service and registering new users would be the main additional responsibilities. There may be no need for additional staff, equipment, or space. Any added duties might be distributed among existing public services staff or given to the circulation department, for example.

More ambitious plans that involve combining access with document delivery, major photocopy center operations, or large-scale document delivery programs which seek a wide user population will not be so easily folded into existing operations. If these services are intended to run on a cost recovery basis, they will need to generate substantial volume. To generate the necessary volume, they will require some dedicated staff, space in which to operate, substantial promotional efforts, record keeping, accounting, and billing; indeed, they will have most of the attributes of a small business. Management of a service of this size and complexity could be added onto an interlibrary loan operation, a circulation department, or another unit in the library; there may be certain advantages in doing this related to economy of scale and per unit cost if use of the new service is expected to be of low volume, particularly during start-up. However, one may also wish to consider some of the advantages to creating a separate department.

One of the chief advantages of creating a separate department for a fee-based service is to improve accountability and financial control. If the financial goal of the service is to recover costs, it is easier to monitor this if the service becomes its own cost center. This simplifies the assignment of both direct and indirect costs and clearly associates revenues with the service. Keeping track of customer orders, assessing response time and quality, and maintaining clearly identifiable accounting and billing will all be enhanced. There may also be advantages in having a separate unit when it comes to conforming to CONTU guidelines on copying materials. It may be easier and more reasonable to maintain separate counts if the fee-based service is clearly distinguished from the library as a whole.

Internal flexibility and control may also be improved by establishing a fee-based service as a separate unit. Particularly during start-up, it is likely that some fine-tuning will be required to make the service run smoothly and efficiently. This tinkering could be disruptive to existing services if the new operation was organized as an add-on, and the older services could suffer from the effect of this continuing change. There are disadvantages to compartmentalization, but one advantage is to isolate problems and have the freedom within bounds to respond to them.

Being a separate unit may help the service develop an identity and make it more visible to both staff and users. Very often this identity will include a distinctive name. Promotion of the service will be aided by this separate identity. It will also make it easier to demarcate the boundaries between new services and old, should this be desirable.

Finally, there is the question of status and the need to demonstrate the importance of a new fee-based service. Adding the service to some existing department may send the wrong message to staff. It is less risky but may set the stage for a tentative effort. Setting up a new department with its own head equal to other department heads and reporting to an appropriate level of the library's administration shows that the library has a substantial commitment to the fee-based service.

Having presented these arguments for a separate unit, it must be recognized that this is not always possible and may not be desirable in many cases. Smaller libraries wishing to establish modest fee-based services can ill afford the dedication of staff and resources needed to make a go of a separate unit. There are also potential problems related to rivalry and morale that may be created by establishing and nourishing a new and distinct unit.

Financial Resources

Many aspects of the financing of fee-based services have been touched upon in this chapter. The principal point to be made is that implementing such services requires adequate start-up funding, especially since it is likely that service volume, and thus income, will initially be low. This funding should at least be sufficient to offset new direct costs, including staffing, associated with the service. This subsidy will need to be budgeted from the library's resources, or a separate budget with its own funding will have to be established. Sources for this additional funding for some services such as document delivery might include various units of the parent institution, particularly those involved in research support. It may be reasonable to attempt to gain a share of overhead money from funded grants, for instance. In a hospital setting, support could be sought from the medical staff organization as well as from the hospital administration.

A start-up budget will almost certainly be larger than the ongoing budget needed to support the fully implemented service. It should also include a contingency fund of 20% to 25% [43]. Every attempt should be made to project the amount of time for which this subsidy will be needed. Monitoring of the service's progress in getting onto its own feet should be continuous, but will certainly focus on the time frame initially set out for the end of subsidized operations.

Subsidies do not always consist of actual funds. The library can also help the service by, in effect, lending it staff, space, equipment, and accounting and billing support. Eventually these are costs which should be recovered, but in the beginning some flexibility can be allowed.

The following items may be considered in developing a budget for fee-based services:

- Consultant
- Staff
- Training
- Travel
- Supplies and materials
- Telephone
- Telecommunications
- Furnishings

- Equipment
- Maintenance
- Software
- Promotion
- Postage
- Fees or deposit accounts (e.g., to online services, interlibrary loan providers, commercial suppliers, or copyright holders)
- Contingency.

Accounting and Billing

It should be expected that the fee-based service will have revenues, even though initially they are not enough to support the operation fully. For that reason an accounting and billing system must be in place at the outset. This system will probably have to conform to the library's existing system and follow rules and procedures set up for the institution as a whole. This conformance may cause problems for the fee-based service because the accounting and billing systems of many institutions, especially academic ones, may not respond well to the needs of a businesslike operation. Fund transfers between units can be difficult, personal billing is often resisted, and the use of credit cards by users may be a new challenge to the system. Institutional accounting and billing systems are built for control, not flexibility. Deposit accounts are often used to get around some of these limitations, but the need to pay in advance for services which are as yet unfamiliar may discourage usage. Library business managers usually are more attuned to spending money than taking in revenues. A great deal of patience and cooperative hard work may be required to iron out some of these difficulties. Eager managers of a new service will have to deal with these problems and attempt to educate everyone about the need to be responsive and user-oriented.

Staffing

Good staff can make or break a new fee-based service, and there can be some special problems associated with staffing a service in its early phases. Whether selecting a service manager from among existing staff or recruiting one from outside, there are qualities that one would like to have present. These are not necessarily qualities that are prevalent among members of the library profession, but they certainly can be found. Despite recent research which found that managers of academic library fee-based services do not exhibit markedly different characteristics from other library managers [44], job descriptions should attempt to describe some singular traits such as willingness to take risks, interest in developing new services, and an entrepreneurial orientation, along with managerial and supervisory experience. Some fee-based services are set up to require that staff bring in the money to pay their own salaries. This requirement is certainly an incentive, but such a condition should be made very clear to prospective employees from the outset.

Does the service manager need to be a librarian? Could business experience be equally valid as a prerequisite? Arguments can be made either way regarding this question. Some experience in the library environment is probably necessary. If the service manager is not a librarian, he or she may have difficulty relating the service to the overall mission of the library. Relationships with other professional staff could also be difficult, and the sense of isolation of the service could be exacerbated.

One of the problems with fee-based document delivery services, especially in their initial phases, is that the flow of orders may not be steady. If the service is experiencing success and receiving many orders, staff may be stretched to the limit in trying to fill them. At other times the business may not come in. An adequate yet flexible staffing level can be a major challenge in any operation. Adding staff is not like turning on the tap since training is required for most jobs if they are to be done correctly. One way to deal with this is to shift staff between the fee-based service and other library operations. Another is to pay couriers and copiers on a piecework basis or to hire contract workers. All of these arrangements may have legal, regulatory, and even ethical drawbacks, but they should at least be considered.

Operating Plan

The type of planning to which an earlier section was devoted is often known as strategic planning. When implementing a fee-based service, it is most helpful to have another kind of plan: an operational plan that will be the blueprint for the service [45]. It should be as specific as possible and should cover the first year of operation. Even a relatively modest service can benefit from having an operational plan that will describe what steps will be followed in implementing the service and serve as a yardstick for measuring progress.

The elements necessary for this plan will include the detailed operating budget, the financial control mechanisms, the staffing plan, the schedule for introducing the various services to be offered, the specific publicity plan, the standards for performance, and the measures of success. Actual operations need to be mapped out. Subsystems and interrelated services should be analyzed and scenarios played out.

One very useful approach for operational planning is the use of the flow chart. A systems analysis technique, flow charting can be an entire discipline of its own, but it need not be overly complicated and can yield some very useful information. It is a way of walking through a process, procedure, or even an entire service on paper. It will graphically depict the flow of work and illustrate decision points, options, subroutines, and points of intersection with elements outside the system. Any gaps in a plan can be very effectively exposed by this technique, and mistakes may be avoided before they happen [46-47].

Legal Issues

The literature on legal issues related to fee-based services should be reviewed, including relevant state laws and court decisions [48]. Librarians are strongly advised to contact their institution's legal counsel to discuss these issues before they begin charging for services.

Nonprofit and Not-for-Profit Status

Profit is not always the motive behind charging fees. Universities, medical centers, and hospitals often have nonprofit or not-for-profit status. Fee-for-service operations pose little threat to such status. These services may simply be acting on behalf of the client to access information or documents in return for a fee to cover some or all of the direct costs involved. However, fee-based service units that intend to recover in excess of direct costs need to construct their price schedules to reflect the parent institutions' attitude toward cost recovery, in order to avoid conflict with their tax status.

Nonprofit institutions are generally exempt from paying federal and state taxes. A fee-based service operating within a nonprofit institution might be considered a separate enterprise. Current law states that nonprofit organizations pay federal taxes on income not directly related to the purpose or mission of the organization [49].

Private Sector Competition

Libraries may have contributed to the emergence of private sector competition through not recognizing or ignoring the needs of affiliated and unaffiliated users. Coupled with new technologies and a host of new electronic information sources which have produced a change in the packaging of information and the methods used to access it, these factors have presented consumers with alternatives to libraries. No longer are researchers dependent on the resources of an individual library and its collection and services.

In the late 1970s, some professionals began leaving the traditional setting of libraries to market their services on a free-lance basis. Librarians with little more than a terminal could provide database searching to business people who did not wish to spend their own time doing traditional research in the library. This change resulted in the development of the new business called information brokering [50].

Partly due to the emergence of personal computers on so many desktops, there has been a new interest by former library-only bibliographic utilities, such as OCLC and RLG, in reaching out to the general public. These vendors are introducing access and end-user products such as document delivery to both the general public and the library's own formerly "closed market" of users. Today's information seeker has a new source of distant suppliers who, for a fee, will serve their needs sometimes more quickly and easily than libraries are able to do. Usually these services accept payment by credit card and often require no prearrangement to obtain services. The availability of such services has opened up a whole new competitive market for the library constituents' dollars.

One further issue related to the provision of information for a fee in competition with the private sector is that there may be laws prohibiting the library from doing so. Many states have statutes which forbid state-supported agencies, units, or institutions from engaging in any activity which threatens the prospects of private businesses. Other laws "forbid publicly funded universities and colleges from offering goods and services except in support of their public service mission" [51]. These laws have been used against fee-based service providers at public universities and may affect publicly funded hospitals as well. They can be particularly problematic if the library is offering service to off-campus or nonprimary users. It would be prudent to check with legal counsel to make sure that a planned fee-based service would not be in conflict with such laws.

Confidentiality

As is the case with most professional-client relationships, confidentiality is an issue in fee-based service provision. Confidentiality of library records is a basic right of users in the United States. The assurance of this right must be addressed in various aspects of fee-based services, including marketing confidentiality. Libraries assume the role of insuring the privacy of any user records in the course of their normal routine, but special attention is needed when accepting the added responsibility of meeting the information needs of fee-based clients.

Clients must have the assurance that their identities will be kept private. All promotional materials should refer to this as a fundamental part of the service that need not be requested specifically by the client. When marketing a service, promotional literature may mention types of clients, for instance law firms, corporations, or drug companies, but specific client names need to be kept confidential unless express permission has been given by the client in advance.

The need for confidentiality must be instilled in all staff when they are trained. Work forms should be kept out of view of other clients or library personnel who do not need to have direct access to them. The service may even disguise client names to outside agencies, including other libraries or document delivery providers, by using client numbers or request numbers.

Special attention needs to be taken when selecting space for locating the service within the library. If customers come on-site, there should be private areas which permit confidential negotiation of information needs.

Guarantees

With the current interest in quality in libraries and the literature, service accountability is a major issue. The existing economy and trends for the future point toward the demand for good value in consumer products and services. As Lunden states, "a fee-based service is a business. The clients have high expectations, they care, and they want quality work" [52].

The quality of information retrieved is in part limited by the clients themselves and how accurately they present their questions and state their needs. Librarians must make sure that they fully understand the client's information needs by adequately clarifying questions or citations with the client. Accuracy at the point of request is necessary to ensure that the correct trail is being taken to answer the customer's need.

Clients will demand that they be satisfied with the integrity of the responses and documents that they receive and that they are provided on a timely basis in accordance with their need. Using interlibrary loan as an example, there is a time lag in fulfilling a request that often affects satisfaction and may even discourage use of the service. As with regular users, librarians need to be explicit with clients to make them aware of both costs and lead time involved in obtaining documents. Accurate representation of the service to the client protects the interests of both the library and the client and promotes satisfaction that a good value has been received at a fair cost.

Fee-based services need to make sure that they have written policies and disclaimers in their contracts, brochures, or the cover pages attached to clients' deliverable products that clearly identify possible sources of error. Some fee-based services have been advised to add "hold-harmless" statements which stress that the service cannot be held accountable for inaccuracies in the information retrieved. To avoid liability, service managers may wish to inquire about error-and-omissions insurance coverage. Up-to-date information on insurance carriers and experiences of libraries carrying such insurance is available from the American Library Association [53].

Copyright

Concerns about copyright are extremely relevant to fee-based services. Each library will need to look at its current procedures for complying with copyright laws and guidelines and make necessary changes or enhancements to take its new role as a fee-based service provider into account. Libraries should also discuss these copyright concerns when they consult with their institution's legal counsel on their plans. Additional information on copyright and fee-based document delivery is available in Chapter 1.

The fee-based service may incorporate its interlibrary loan statistics with those of the general requests of the library. In fact, this may occur through default since it is often more cost effective to have one document delivery unit within a library which would handle all such requests, regardless if generated by the fee-based service or regular library users.

However, a separate fee-based service, or even one attached to the library's interlibrary loan department, need not necessarily combine all borrowing statistics for the purpose of following CONTU guidelines. It may be advisable for the fee-based service to keep its business distinct from that of the library and pay Copyright Clearance Center fees on all documents obtained for nonprimary users. This practice will prevent the fee-based service from running up the counts on titles to the detriment of the library and its primary users.

The cost of copyright compliance must be accounted for in determining document delivery costs. Two different methods can be used in connection with these copyright costs. One method is to add a flat copyright fee based upon the average fee incurred. Another is to pass on the exact fee involved with each request to the client. This second method can be difficult when costs may not be known with certainty by the date of delivery to the client. Whatever course is followed, all associated costs need to be addressed and tracked for billing to the client.

Marketing Fee-Based Services

Librarians grappling with the issue of marketing and promotion can seek some help from the business literature about the topic. Many business-related sources have a wealth of information, but sources listed in the references are specific to the topic in respect to libraries [54-59]. Examples of promotional materials from library fee-based services are included in *The FISCAL Primer*, materials compiled by the ACRL discussion group FISCAL that is available at cost from the Coordinator, Gelman Library Information Service, George Washington University, 2130 H Street NW, Room B07, Washington DC 20052 [60].

Pricing Strategies

The pricing of products and services relates to the earlier discussion of financial models and policies involved in setting prices. The marketing, business, and library literatures provide greater detail on pricing strategies for both the profit and nonprofit sectors [61-62]. The following will briefly discuss some of the major points.

There are three primary pricing strategies: cost-based, demand-based, and competition-based [63-64]. Selection of a pricing strategy follows the establishment of pricing objectives. Cost-based pricing primarily establishes charges relative to expenses incurred. Full-cost pricing is the most common form found in the nonprofit sector and is determined by the addition of all direct and indirect costs. A variety of cost-based pricing strategies are available. Full and partial-cost recovery are fairly self-explanatory. Cost-plus pricing adds a fixed percentage on top of the cost of a job. Similarly, target rate of return, markup, and value-added pricing use various approaches to add on fixed or variable charges in addition to the actual costs involved in providing the product or service. Token, loss-leader, and minimum-value pricing are essentially promotional pricing strategies that settle for less than cost recovery for some part of a service or product with the intention of making up the loss on other parts.

Demand-based pricing gives primary consideration to demand, rather than costs, in establishing prices. This pricing formula charges what the market will bear. The price for a product or service should reflect the value that the client perceives it is worth. With demand-based pricing, prices are lowered with weak demand and increased with high demand. Demand-based pricing is frequently a form of discriminatory pricing for services which are offered to different markets, such as document delivery for affiliated versus unaffiliated users. Primary users may be charged the direct variable cost incurred from a document supplier, while nonaffiliated users may be charged a higher rate per article to cover total costs. To implement demand-based pricing effectively, service managers will need to exploit their market research to assess what services or products should be offered, to whom, how, and at what cost.

Competition-based pricing is determined by what other information providers are charging for similar products or services. Libraries new to the fee-based service arena are usually interested in finding out what other fee-based services are charging, hoping to receive guidance in setting their own prices. However, the prices charged by other services should not be the principal element in the formulation of a pricing structure. A favorite form of competitive strategy is imitative pricing, where the prices match or attempt to undercut those that major competitors are charging. This strategy is seen quite frequently in the business world.

Fees should be reviewed periodically to reexamine pricing objectives and strategies and to determine if changes need to be made. Prices normally go up as costs of a service increase with time, although, rarely, costs and prices do come down. When costs decrease, it is likely due to increased efficiency or economies of scale which can be realized as a service matures. Usually when prices change, there is a corresponding change in demand for services, but in most instances the demand level stabilizes after a period of adjustment by the customer.

Promotion

Fee-based services must make use of communication as a marketing tool. There are essentially two types of promotion, each of which needs to be incorporated into any fee-based program: indirect and direct marketing communications. Each has a place within the total marketing plan and enables the service to take advantage of opportunities to stress the benefits of using the services offered. Although some strategies require the commitment of significant financial resources, others can be undertaken on a low budget.

Indirect marketing communications are broad, general attention grabbers. Sometimes called venture marketing, these strategies are aimed at the total market or large specific market sectors with many prospects. The major tools include overall public relations, printed marketing tools, advertising, and exhibiting and speaking. Direct marketing, on the other hand, is client-oriented to particular smaller segments of the market, showing how the service will solve particular problems or answer individual needs. Communications are very specific and tailored messages in areas of interest to potential customers. Communications may be to individuals or groups, but they are always directed toward specific prospects. Examples of direct marketing include such things as direct mail, focused presentations, video-tapes, and project reports.

The public relations department of a hospital or university can be of great help in promoting a fee-based service. It may provide assistance in preparing press releases, designing brochures, writing articles about the service, and including articles in hospital or university publications and other promotional items.

Press releases or stories for area newsletters can be effective promotional tools that cost very little. Inclusion of this type of material in an area medical society newsletter or journal will bring the service to the attention of physicians. Since small publications eagerly seek contributions, this method of promotion provides large exposure at limited cost. Copies or reprints of any articles should be obtained by the service for use in related marketing efforts and to serve as a promotional archive.

A brochure, which can be used in many ways, is probably essential (Figure 4-1). A successful brochure will gain the attention of prospects if it contains useful information and provokes interest. It should include complete information on the service, how to contact it and who is eligible, fees and billing, and statements on guarantees and liability. A separate insert for prices, which can be more frequently updated and reprinted, is recommended. It is helpful to stress the benefits of the service: what clients may ask for and specific problems the service can solve. A checklist of items to include in a brochure is available in Warner [65].

Good brochures are difficult to write and to design. Initially the fee-based staff should work on the draft of a brochure because they know the services best. The copy should be reviewed by persons outside the profession, preferably potential clients, in addition to other staff. It can be a challenge to represent ideas and concepts in terms that will be understood by the general audience for whom the material is intended. It must guard against the tendency to speak to other librarians instead of clients; as with all library materials, services should be described in clear simple terms, avoiding library jargon. After a preliminary brochure is developed, it should be produced using desktop publishing software or submitted to a layout artist with experience in the production of publicity brochures.

A newsletter or regular publication from the library can be an effective promotional strategy. It not only may serve as a vehicle to announce the service but also may convey changes and improvement to services or highlight milestones of success. Newsletters distributed to individuals in the institution serve as a constant reminder of the library and inform individuals of the services available.

An annual report for the fee-based service can be published to promote services. Examples of the kinds of information requests may be given, with descriptions of the delivered responses from the service. Graphs may be

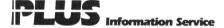

PLUS is the UCSD Library's information service for San Diego businesses, professionals, government agencies, and community members.

PLUS is a one-stop information provider— a telephone call, electronic mail message, telefacsimile, or visit initiates your information request.

PLUS finds the information you need by connecting to electronic networks and databases that access global information sources.

PLUS obtains materials worldwide to answer your questions.

PLUS provides fast, accurate information at a reasonable price.

PLUS is a customized service—you pay for what you need.

PLUS is confidential.

Figure 4-1: Inner Panels of Sample Brochure (Panel 1)
(Reproduced with permission of Corporate Programs Office, University of California, San Diego Libraries)

PLUS provides...

Document Services

- Photocopies of articles
- UCSD library cards
- Materials borrowed from other libraries
- Materials obtained from other sources

Research

- Searches in online databases, printed indexes, government, business, and industrial information sources to answer your questions.
- In-depth customized reports are available.

Information Tracking

- Access to over 200 commercial databases including science, engineering, medicine, business and government information.

  Staff regularly scan databases to monitor your specific area of interest and send you a list of the latest articles and reports covering your subject.

Document Delivery

- Photocopies, materials borrowed from other libraries, information tracking lists, and reports are delivered via mail, telefacsimile, Federal Express, UPS, or special courier.

PLUS locates information on...

- State-of-the-art technology
- Standards and specifications
- Research in progress
- Patents/trademarks
- Government regulations

  - Marketing statistics
  - Economic forecasts
  - Company information
  - Trade news
  - Competitor activities
  - Industry outlook

- Names and addresses
- Biographical data
- Lists of manufacturers
- Technical data

Figure 4-1: (Panel 2)

PLUS delivers...

- Books
- Journal articles
- Technical reports
- Government documents
- Conference papers

PLUS provides...

- A competitive edge by supplying you with the latest information in your field.

- Global information coverage through online and printed sources.

- Access to libraries nationwide.

- Referrals to alternate sources.

- Professional research librarians who work with you to answer your questions quickly, accurately, and confidentially.

- Time savings—a telephone call, telefacsimile, or electronic mail message requests information services—you don't have to spend time in the library.

PLUS staff bring information resources – online and print – directly to you.

Figure 4-1: (Panel 3)

used to show the client breakdown by industry sectors or the number of documents provided. Photographs showing staff at work and brief staff biographies can provide human interest.

Advertising is an expensive and risky avenue to gain exposure that appears not to have worked very well for most fee-based services. If a fee-based service elects to try this form of promotion, it is strongly advised that experienced help be solicited to write and design advertisements and position them in the most suitable places and publications. Sometimes local newspapers will run supplements on topics that may be appropriate for advertising health-related information services. Taking out advertising space in membership directories of professional associations in the surrounding communities and in their journals, newsletters, and various publications can be effective. An example would be the local bar association newsletter or a journal that is read by the legal community, who is often interested in obtaining medical information but may have limited expertise. Mixed success has been found with listings in the classified section of the telephone directory; determining how to list a service for which there is no standardization of terms and an audience which may be unfamiliar with where to look are deterrents. If advertising is used, records should be kept on the number of clients generated by each effort.

Exhibiting at professional association meetings may be another way to reach new customers. Exhibits permit personal communication, the single most effective method of promoting the advantages of the service and stimulating a desire for a product. Innovative and creative media such as a video or slide/tape program can orient attendees to products and services. Brochures, fact sheets, and business cards should be available. Whoever staffs a booth must have a clear understanding of all particulars of the service and have an outgoing energetic presence. It is advisable to discuss this type of promotion with those who have experience and may offer assistance in preparation. Although an expensive and time-consuming activity, exhibiting can be most beneficial to new services in attracting clients.

It is useful for a service manager to be a good public speaker. Many opportunities exist for presentations at institutional or area meetings. The hospital public relations or university alumni office should be made aware of the manager's availability to speak.

Because of its success in business, direct mail advertising is growing faster than any other type of marketing; however it is fairly new to the library setting [66]. A market strategy is established which identifies the needs and wants of a selected group and then matches them with specific library services. The personalized nature of direct mail targets individuals with common characteristics. A printed piece such as a letter, brochure, or return postcard is sent to prospects who are perceived to be potential clients. The literature states that direct mail as a general rule will yield a 1 to 1.5% client generation rate, that is, a mailing to 1,000 appropriate prospects will generate ten to fifteen new clients [67]. What mailing list to use will depend on whom the fee-based service has targeted. Lists may be available from in-house sources such as the human resources department or public relations department. Mailing list catalogs can also be obtained from list brokers who, for a fee, will provide preprinted name and address labels.

Ultimately the best promotion is satisfied customers. Word-of-mouth advertising cannot be overlooked or overvalued. All the good efforts of marketing and promotion can be wiped away by a few dissatisfied customers. Bad news travels fast, and disgruntled clients are likely to be vocal and share their complaints with others. Satisfied clients are also a good source of material for written promotion; testimonials and quotations should be documented and collected for future use.

Image

Image is a cornerstone to fee-based service marketing strategies. How a service is perceived by the public and potential clients is important to the success of any service. It is imperative that each staff member remember that every person who uses or visits the service is a potential messenger of goodwill or a possible new client. They need to be assured that they are choosing a service that will not only meet their needs, but one which presents a professional image that inspires confidence.

A service should take advantage of its affiliation with a reputable hospital or university. This reputation has likely taken years to develop and will convey integrity, permanence, and excellence backed up with a wide range of resources. The library itself very likely possesses extensive resources and collection strengths and its own good reputation for quality services.

The name of a fee-based service is yet another aspect of the overall image of the service. Selection of a name may take into account the products of the service and the library in which the service is housed. It should be easy to remember and allow the flexibility to expand the scope of the service.

Fee-based service staff need to build a reputation for themselves, taking every opportunity to gain exposure through networking and to maintain a high visibility with colleagues and potential clients. Becoming involved with trade and professional associations and societies is one way to work towards this goal.

Appearance is important in maintaining and promoting a professional image. A businesslike attitude is necessary in all aspects of the fee-based service. It is not the place to project a relaxed collegiate image. Professional attire is critical to working with clients. Time and effort should be taken in the choice and design of business cards, stationery, and correspondence. The confidence of clients that they have made the right choice in selecting a service may be bolstered by seeing that the staff of the service take their work seriously.

Evaluation

Day-to-day operations can be all-consuming when beginning a fee-based service. It is very easy to become buried in the regular flow of work and to forget about the original plans that were written to guide the smooth implementation of the service. Baseline data should be gathered at the beginning of the service implementation so as to determine if the service is growing and prospering as planned. Careful tracking of costs should be done to assess the balance between revenues generated and expenses incurred. The original planning documents need to be revisited and comparisons made between projections and what is really happening. Adaptation may be necessary once the service has had time to get underway.

As with any new business venture, progress needs to be monitored as the business begins to grow and develop. The current operating plan should be reviewed on an ongoing basis. Workflow, staffing levels, and output should be analyzed if problems have emerged that cause delays in delivery or impede sales. The budget will need close review to see if anticipated revenue is indeed covering expenses. If not, planned expenses may need to be postponed until revenues improve or additional support is obtained. There are many existing software packages for all types of personal computers which will assist with project management and track goals and timeframes. In the early stages of a business, flexibility and a close eye on potential problems are mandatory; they are perhaps more important than strictly following a strategic plan.

Making sure that clients are getting what they have paid for should be addressed as part of the evaluative process for a fee-based service. Establishing performance standards can help to insure that good service is provided to all clients. In addition, user feedback should be sought to assure that expectations are being met. It is very important that all staff have a clear understanding of written performance and service standards. Staff should be active participants in developing such standards. Their ideas for improving processes and thereby providing better service should also be encouraged.

Conclusion

Fee-based services in libraries of all types will continue to be controversial as long as the strongly held value favoring free and equal access to information continues to be endorsed by the profession. At the same time, pressures on libraries, pressures which perhaps threaten the very existence of these institutions as they currently operate, are predicted to continue to grow. These include competition for the resources of the parent institutions of libraries, competition from nonlibrary information purveyors, and competition among stronger and weaker libraries themselves.

Matheson warns that most of today's libraries cannot survive as libraries of the future. Some will continue as "just-in-case" libraries, continuing to amass or hold onto traditional resources so that the "just-in-time" libraries can operate. Others will move to developing and owning new digital knowledge resources and to making these accessible. Still a third group will survive by knowing where knowledge is and how to mine it [68]. While Matheson did not say so, it is possible that these scenarios will be heavily dependent on fee-based components. Certainly any one of them could follow a fee-based model.

In fact, there are those who feel that nonlibrary competitors will continue to break off pieces of the library's function and market services to those potential library users who are most able to pay, leaving moribund those libraries which fail to adapt. The advice of people such as Kuenzle is that every library which wishes to survive should find some way to develop a fee-based service [69]. Whether this is a realistic admonition or not, it seems certain that the economic and information environment of the future will force many libraries to at least consider doing just that.

References

1. Josephine H. Fee-based services in ARL libraries. Washington, DC: Association of Research Libraries, Office of Management Services, September 1989. (SPEC flyer 157).

2. Nshaiwat NAM. Issues in fee-based information service in academic libraries: entrepreneurial characteristics and managerial activities [dissertation]. [Bloomington]: Indiana University, 1989:8.

3. Downing A. The consequences of offering fee-based services in a medical library. Bull Med Libr Assoc 1990 Jan; 78(1):57-63.

4. Foreman GE. Fee-for-service in publicly supported libraries: an overview. In: Wood MS, ed. Cost analysis, cost recovery, marketing, and fee-based services: a guide for the health sciences librarian. New York: Haworth Press, 1985:175-83.

5. Coffman S, Josephine H. Doing it for money. Libr J 1991 Oct; 116(17):32-3.

6. Roche MM. ARL/RLG interlibrary loan cost study: a joint effort by the Association of Research Libraries and the Research Libraries Group. Washington, DC: Association of Research Libraries, 1993.

7. ALA policy manual 1.2-1.3. In: ALA handbook of organization. Chicago: American Library Association, 1992:133-4.

8. Lyders RA. Task force drafts ethics code. MLA News 1994 Mar;(263):1,7.

9. ALA policy manual 50.4. In: ALA handbook of organization. Chicago: American Library Association, 1992:144.

10. Giacoma P. The fee or free decision: legal, economic, political, and ethical perspectives for public libraries. New York: Neal-Schuman, 1989:161-75.

11. Ibid., 86.

12. FISCAL (Fee-Based Information Service Centers in Academic Libraries). FISCAL primer [Compilation of materials on topic].

13. Dearie TN, Steel V. Interlibrary loan trends: making access a reality. Washington, DC: Association of Research Libraries, Office of Management Services, 1992. (SPEC flyer 184).

14. Conference on fee-based research in college and university libraries: proceedings of the meetings at C. W. Post Center of Long Island University, Greenvale, New York, June 17-18, 1982, sponsored by the Center for Business Research and the B. Davis Schwartz Memorial Library at the C. W. Post Center of Long Island University. Greenvale, NY: The Center, 1983.

15. Nshaiwat, op. cit., 6.

16. Josephine, op. cit.

17. FISCAL, op. cit.

18. Bunting A. The nation's health information network: history of the Regional Medical Library Program, 1965 1985. Bull Med Libr Assoc 1987 July;75(Suppl 3):1-62.

19. Williams TL, Lemkau HL, Burrows S. The economics of academic health sciences libraries: cost recovery in the era of big science. Bull Med Libr Assoc 1988 Oct;76(4):317-22.

20. Bloomquist H, Rees AM, Stearns NS, Yast H, eds. Library practice in hospitals: a basic guide. Cleveland: Case Western Reserve University, 1972.

21. Wakeley PJ, Bayorgeon M. Interlibrary loan. In: Bradley J, Holst R, Messerle J, eds. Hospital library management. Chicago: Medical Library Association, 1983:145-62.

22. Messerle J. Information services. In: Bradley J, Holst R, Messerle J, eds. Hospital library management. Chicago: Medical Library Association, 1983:104-24.

23. Jones CL, Kasses CD. Lending services: circulation policies, procedures, and problems. In: Darling L, Bishop D, Colaianni LA, eds. Handbook of medical library practice. 4th ed. v.1. Chicago: Medical Library Association, 1982:65-94.

24. Middleton DR. Lending services: interlibrary loan/document delivery. In: Darling L, Bishop D, Colaianni LA, eds. Handbook of medical library practice. 4th ed. v.1. Chicago: Medical Library Association, 1982:95-136.

25. McClure L. Reference services: policies and practices. In: Darling L, Bishop D, Colaianni LA, eds. Handbook of medical library practice. 4th ed. v.1. Chicago: Medical Library Association, 1982:137-81.

26. Egeland J, Foreman G. Reference services: searching and search techniques. In: Darling L, Bishop D, Colaianni LA, eds. Handbook of medical library practice. 4th ed. v.1. Chicago: Medical Library Association, 1982:183-235.

27. Werner G. Use of on-line bibliographic retrieval services in health sciences libraries in the United States and Canada. Bull Med Libr Assoc 1979 Jan;67(1):1-15.

28. Wood SM, ed. Cost analysis, cost recovery, marketing, and fee-based services: a guide for the health sciences librarian. New York: Haworth Press, 1985.

29. Drucker P. Management: tasks, responsibilities, practices. New York: Harper & Row, 1974:512.

30. Cargill J, Webb GM. Managing libraries in transition. Phoenix, AZ: Oryx Press, 1988:82.

31. Warner AS. Making money: fees for library services. New York: Neal-Schuman, 1989:7-8.

32. Coffman S, Wildensohler P. The FISCAL directory of fee-based research and document supply services. 4th ed. Los Angeles: County of Los Angeles Public Library, 1993.

33. Josephine, op. cit., 2.

34. Barrett GJ. The costs of interlibrary loan. ARL 1993 Jan;166:1-2.

35. Warner, op. cit., 45-7.

36. Stump B. Operating and marketing fee-based services in academic libraries: a small business approach. [Chicago]: Association of College and Research Libraries, 1983:14-5. (ACRL continuing education program CE 108a).

37. Ferber R, ed. Handbook of marketing research. New York: McGraw-Hill, 1974.

38. Warner, op. cit.

39. Lemkau HL, Burrows S, La Rocco A. Marketing information services outside the medical center. In: Wood SM, ed. Cost analysis, cost recovery, marketing, and fee-based services: a guide for the health sciences librarian. New York: Haworth Press, 1985:143-57.

40. Dillman DA. Mail and telephone surveys: the total design method. New York: Wiley, 1978.

41. Stewart DW. Focus groups: theory and practice. Newburg Park, CA: Sage Publications, 1990.

42. Herman L. Costing, charging, and pricing; related but different decisions. Bottom Line 1990 Summer;4(2):26-8.

43. Warner, op. cit., 62.

44. Nshaiwat, op. cit., 136-41.

45. Stump, op. cit., 17D-E.

46. Wetherbe JC. Systems analysis and design. St. Paul, MN: West Publishing, 1988.

47. Chapman EA. Systems analysis and design as related to library operations; a manual for a symposium sponsored by the Upstate New York Chapter, Special Libraries Association, Saratoga Springs, N.Y., September 17-18, 1966. Troy, NY: Rensselaer Libraries, 1966.

48. Wood WD. A librarian's guide to fee-based services. Ref Libr 1993;(40):121-9.

49. Warner, op. cit., 75.

50. Kinder R, Katz B. Information brokers and reference services. New York: Haworth Press, 1988.

51. Goldberg B. University's library fee-service upheld. Am Libr 1989 Mar;20(3):188.

52. Lunden E. The library as business. Am Libr 1982 Jul/Aug;13(7):471-2.

53. Warner, op. cit., 73-4.

54. MLS (Marketing library service), v.1, 1987- .

55. Marketing treasures, v.1, 1987- .

56. Schmidt J. Marketing the modern information center: a guide to intrapreneurship for the information manager. New York: FIND/SVP, 1987.

57. Walters S. Marketing: a how-to-do-it manual for librarians. New York: Neal-Schuman, 1992. (How-to-do-it manuals for libraries no. 20).

58. Wood EJ. Strategic marketing for libraries: a handbook. New York: Greenwood Press, 1988.

59. Weingand DE. Marketing/planning library and information services. Littleton, CO: Libraries Unlimited, 1987.

60. FISCAL, op. cit.

61. Jacob MEL. Costing and pricing: the difference matters. Bottom Line 1988;2(2):12-4.

62. Virgo JAC. Costing and pricing information services. In: Cronin B, ed. The marketing of library and information services 2. London: Aslib, 1992:259-78.

63. Zais HW. Economic modeling: an aid to the pricing of information services. J Am Soc Inf Sci 1977 Mar;28(2):89-95.

64. Kibirige HM. The information dilemma: a critical analysis of information pricing and the fees controversy. Westport, CT: Greenwood Press, 1983: 105-18. (New directions in librarianship no. 4).

65. Warner, op. cit., 122-3.

66. Tepper K. Direct mail advertising: a library application. Unabashed Libr 1989;(73):13-5.

67. Warner, op. cit., 132.

68. Matheson NW. The idea of the library in the twenty-first century. Bull Med Libr Assoc 1995 Jan;83(1):1-7.

69. Kuenzle D. Change, chance and the challenge. Keynote address. Presented at the Annual meeting of the Mid-Atlantic Chapter, Medical Library Association, Asheville, NC, October 6, 1994.

5

Future Trends

Beryl Glitz and Irene Lovas

Information access and delivery can perhaps be described as the "bottom line" for libraries. No matter how sophisticated the bibliographic control or how comprehensive the collection, to satisfy its users a library must be able to deliver the actual information, whatever the format, into the users' hands. While traditionally this has meant that library users needed to go to the library for the information, today, more and more, the trend is for the information to go to the users. Technology has been the key to this shift. With technology, new methods have been developed that reduce the time needed for information access and delivery and increase both the variety of resources available and the ways to deliver them, often without users having to set foot into the actual library or to interact with library staff [1]. This technology is beginning to have a significant impact on library operations and budgets, especially in the areas of circulation and interlibrary loan.

In this chapter, the focus is on how technology has changed the way users get access to the information they seek and the way that information is delivered to them, either directly by the local library or through the resources of other libraries or commercial providers. While all aspects in the continuum of access and delivery have been affected by technological advances, it is in the areas of document delivery and interlibrary lending that the most changes have occurred. New systems are continually being developed that take advantage of the increasing capabilities of telecommunications and digital storage. These systems not only improve the speed of information delivery, they indeed change the very nature of the information delivered. This chapter will look at several of these systems and their effects on library operations; it also will consider the implications that these effects will have in the future on the traditional roles the library has played in the access and delivery of information. Also discussed will be several related issues affected by this shift, including copyright, licensing, staff training, and the changing balance between access and ownership of library materials. Just what these continuing trends might mean to the library community will be explored.

Traditional Access and Delivery

For centuries, seekers of information have come to the library in the expectation that what they hope to find will be there. The library, for its part, has responded to this expectation with a variety of services and systems which have changed little for many years. First, the library catalog, whether in book, card, or more recently online format, tells users if the library owns a particular piece of information. Though larger libraries will usually have catalogs that list both books and journals, smaller libraries may maintain separate journal listings. Whether integrated or separate, these resources located within the library will provide the details, usually a call number or shelving location, so that users can retrieve the needed information from the shelf.

Secondly, the arrangement of the collections, usually by call number for books or alphabetically by title for journals, permits users to go directly to the item required, or if the library has closed stacks, a paging service brings the item to the users. Thirdly, a circulation system, which uniquely identifies both the items and the users, allows users to check out the information they need to use either at home, in the laboratory, or in the office. Such a system, whether card or computer-based, enables the library to keep track of where circulating items are and when they are due back. The system also allows for items to be recalled if requested by another user and for the loan period to be extended through a renewal, usually made in-person or over the telephone. In some health sciences libraries, where institutional staff have access to the library after regular hours, circulation systems can be simple enough to allow users to check out the items when library staff are not available.

A fourth and final service to deliver library information to users is the photocopy machine. Whether providing for self-service copying or a document delivery service managed by library staff, the photocopy machine has long been a library staple. This is especially true in the health sciences where so much of the information needed is found in journal articles and where journal collections of many institutions do not circulate.

If the needed item is on the library shelf, these methods work together to provide users with rapid access and delivery. The library has also developed systems for access and delivery when the needed item is not readily available in the local collection. Referred to traditionally as interlibrary loan (ILL), this service draws on the collections of other libraries to fill requests which the user's library does not own. Based on reciprocal agreements between libraries throughout the country, and indeed throughout the world, ILL service has been an important and labor-intensive function of libraries for many years. In health sciences libraries particularly, the ILL network is highly developed because of the speed with which much patient-related information is needed. Once it has been determined, usually by trained library staff, that a needed item is not owned locally, a complex series of procedures swing into action to track down, request, and deliver that item. Such procedures, using local and networked systems, are in place in almost every library. With the necessary bibliographic information and details about the requester, library staff can apply these procedures, using a host of resources, union catalogs, and online systems such as OCLC or DOCLINE. When the item arrives, the borrowing library will either mail the item to the requester or send a notice that the item is ready for pickup. While traditional delivery patterns have usually been through the mail or private courier, telefacsimile machines have been a welcome addition to these methods, especially in the health care field where speed is often, literally, a matter of life and death.

Whether items are taken off the shelf by the users, paged by the library staff, photocopied, checked out, or delivered from another collection, the traditional model for information access and delivery has always depended on users coming to the library and upon the intervention of trained library staff performing various library functions: circulation, reference, and ILL. With the development of a variety of computerized systems and telecommunications capabilities, this traditional model has been steadily changing.

Remote Access to and Delivery of Local Resources

Recent Advances

In the past decade many libraries, including those in the health sciences, have begun to develop a "library without walls" so that users can perform many of the functions which traditionally required a trip to the library from their offices, off-site clinics, or homes. Without leaving home or the workplace, users can now determine if their library has an item needed to diagnose a difficult case or to verify results for a research project. They can then electronically request delivery of that item, have it recalled if circulating to another user, or request that the item be obtained from another library if it is not in the collection. If users already have an item which they need to keep longer, they can electronically request a renewal; there is no need to make trips or telephone calls to the library.

Several developments have made these types of remote access possible. One major factor has been the spread of personal computers into offices, clinics, laboratories, and homes. While they may have been introduced initially for word processing or other office management procedures, the addition of a modem or fax-modem, telephone hookup and, more recently, the direct linking to a local computer or network, have greatly extended the functions of these workstations. A second factor in providing remote access has been the widespread development of machine-readable databases of bibliographic records. Individual libraries, government agencies, and commercial and not-for-profit institutions have all been involved in this pursuit. Concentrating initially on the journal literature, many of these databases have been mounted and made available by commercial enterprises. Online public access catalogs (OPACs) now provide millions of machine-readable records for a variety of library materials, including books, journals, and audiovisuals [2]. A third and final development critical to the provision of remote access has been the creation of computer networks. Connected through the telephone line or hardwired throughout an institution or campus, these networks have created the link between the user's local workstation and the various online information resources.

While much of this activity has taken place on large university campuses, in the health sciences arena a concerted effort has been made by libraries, beginning in the early 1980s, to enhance access to their services, saving both users and institutions time and money. In 1982, the Matheson-Cooper report, *Academic Information in the Academic Health Sciences Center* [3], provided perhaps the best description of the technological applications that would affect the access to and delivery of information to library users. One of the goals expressed in this report was to bridge "the gap between the user and the information wanted by making the transfer of information through multiple (computer) systems both rapid and practical" [4].

Many academic health sciences libraries in the spirit of the Matheson report have used their campus-wide network to provide expanded access to library services. At the University of Tennessee at Memphis, for example, as in many academic medical centers, users can currently request library services by electronic mail rather than by the more traditional methods [5]. They can complete forms on a computer screen, rather than use paper forms, to request photocopies of journal articles or ILLs and to renew circulating items. The users then need only to come to the library to pick up the requested items which are waiting for them. They also can find out about library hours and services without going to the library or telephoning. Having this remote access twenty-four hours a day makes the library resources available to all users at all times. This access to the library supplements in-house library use. "Instead of the library disappearing with the emergence of electronic information, it becomes just another node in the . . . user's information network" [6].

While such systems have expanded the services of the library enormously and provided information access to library users where they most needed it, the library's information has until recently always been stored separately from other online data that might exist in an institution. Emphasizing the importance of integrating information from all sources in a hospital or academic setting, the National Library of Medicine (NLM) has been instrumental over the past ten years in supporting and funding the concept of Integrated Advanced Information Management Systems (IAIMS). NLM has long been concerned with how to meet the information needs of health professionals in the emerging era of high technology and has strongly advocated that libraries be the leaders in supporting the development of information network systems [7].

An IAIMS grant program was initiated in 1984 to assist institutions in developing integrated information systems to link the resources of the library to the functions of a medical center. While most of the institutions awarded IAIMS grants have been academic medical centers, many hospitals have developed similar information systems connecting various patient care departments such as patient records; departments specializing in clinical diagnosis, such as the laboratory, pathology, and radiology; appointment scheduling; and information systems, including the library. At Columbia-Presbyterian Medical Center, one of the institutions awarded an IAIMS grant from NLM, the goal was "to provide access from a single workstation to clinical, research, and library resources," thus creating a "common network of access and delivery" [8]. As part of the Columbia-Presbyterian and other network systems, users can select from a menu screen various library components and request literature searches, browse the library's computerized catalog and serials list, request items from the library's collection, renew materials, and request ILLs for items not in the collection. A further development has been the mounting of an electronic textbook onto the system, thus providing a new kind of access to the full text of library materials rather than just the bibliographic information. The library also can communicate electronically with users to inform them about the status of their requests. Through the information system, users receive notification about items to be picked up or ones that are overdue. The users then must go to the library to pick up the requests if they are not delivered by courier, mail, fax, or other traditional methods.

Agencies other than NLM are also encouraging this movement toward the integration of all types of information vital to a hospital or medical center. Beginning with the 1994 standards, the Joint Commission on Accreditation of Healthcare Organizations (JCAHO) completed the first of two phases which will transform the organization of their standards from one based on hospital departments or services to one based on functions critical to patient care. The former section "Professional Library and Health Information Services" has been incorporated as part of the function of management of information, which is to obtain, manage, and use information to improve an organization's performance in the areas of patient care, governance, and management. The section, now entitled "Knowledge-Based Information," relates most directly to the changing functions of the library. Knowledge-based information also can be referred to as the "literature," and its management provides for identifying, organizing, retrieving, analyzing, delivering, and reporting clinical and managerial journal literature, reference information, and research data as they are used to design, manage, and improve patient-specific and organizational processes. As hospital administrators now plan to meet the new standards for managing information, they will assess the following needs for knowledge-based information: accessibility and timeliness, linkages with the organization's internal information systems, and linkages with appropriate external databases and networks [9]. Since organizations will have up to five years to achieve these information management standards, an increase in more hospital-wide information systems which include the library can be expected.

Clearly these integrated systems have greatly improved communication with the library and easy access to information about its books and journals. Requesting and receiving the actual documents is, however, still a problem for library users, since in many systems these functions remain very much rooted in tradition, and library staff must intervene to procure items through regular ILL procedures. There are, however, some developments using technological advancements that place the requesting of items, whether locally available or at distant sites, in the hands of the users. One such system is ORION EXPRESS at the University of California, Los Angeles (UCLA) Louise Darling Biomedical Library. The service allows for initial online registration of users and subsequent ordering of journal articles directly from the online catalog record. Requested items are then mailed to campus addresses or picked up by off-campus users. While available only for journal requests initially, the service has since been expanded to include books. At the University of Oregon, two different online services are provided for registered users to order journal articles. A photocopy service allows users to place orders for individual journal articles retrieved from a search of the library's MEDLINE subset. The orders are then downloaded and filled by the library, and the users' orders are acknowledged online. Another feature of the Oregon system is REQUESTLINE which allows users to upload a group of requests simultaneously from a monthly SDI update performed by library staff searchers. Articles requested by either service can be mailed or picked up by requesters.

Future Trends

With few exceptions, the type of remote access described in the previous section has been to the traditional bibliographic information that libraries have always provided to their users. Along with these descriptions of library materials, however, some of the remote systems are also including the capability for users to request electronically the actual materials listed. A further development along these lines, as seen at Columbia-Presbyterian, is to provide online access to the complete text of the actual materials.

Full-text access to some journal articles has been available for several years through commercial online systems. The InfoPro Technologies (formerly BRS) service, CCML (Comprehensive Core Medical Library), is one example, providing the text of a limited number of medical journals to any code-holder for searching and printing. With the recent development of several electronic journals, some with more sophisticated search capabilities, the full contents of the recent journal literature may become more widely available online, though at present full-text access overall is to just a small percentage of the entire biomedical literature. The mounting of full text by libraries is, however, something new and could provide a tremendous service to users, while reducing the library's need to purchase subscriptions and to bind and shelve volumes. Staff time for checking-in and tracking the issues also would be reduced. In a survey by the Association of Research Libraries, 42% of the responding libraries were involved in some type of text digitization, for storage, retrieval, or dissemination [10]. A few libraries, such as those at North Carolina State University and Virginia Polytechnic University, are beginning to develop their own electronic journals, but very few are in the process of creating online books. The number of books available as full-text files from commercial publishers is also small, though increasing, but it is unlikely that commercial enterprises will go back and retrospectively convert older materials. Does the library have a role here? With dwindling space and smaller book budgets, electronic rather than physical access might be a viable alternative, especially if embarked on cooperatively by a group of libraries. Once the necessary equipment and communication channels are in place and the copyright and ownership issues resolved, libraries might well choose to create their own online books and other types of materials. Academic institutions, for example, might find it cost-effective to create such items as course syllabi or composite textbooks. The class reserve readings which must now be laboriously copied, filed, and then removed at the end of each academic session would be ready candidates for this type of storage and access.

Ease of access, lack of money, and diminishing storage space are all strong incentives for libraries to provide more and more information in online format, whether developed commercially or through their own efforts. Coupled with recent advances in computer software such as XWindows, libraries are beginning to realize the concept of the "scholarly workstation," where the individual researcher can have instant and seamless access to a world of information that can be manipulated and introduced into the user's working environment.

A recent collaboration is a good example of the type of service a library might provide to its users in the future. Red Sage, a research project underway at the Library at the University of California, San Francisco (UCSF), is experimenting with providing online access to Springer-Verlag journals in radiology and molecular biology. The project seeks to make the online journals look and feel as much like paper products as possible. Using software developed by Bell Laboratories, each article is stored as a text file, while each page of the article is also saved as a photographic image, including all the illustrations exactly as they appear on paper. The system was initially developed on a UNIX workstation but is also useable on both Macintosh and IBM machines and includes full-color illustrations. A highlight of this project is the added features being developed which will provide an array of information services, all available from the same workstation. An alerting function now sends automatic e-mail messages to any user who has stored a subject interest profile on the system whenever an article of interest is added. A search program will allow users to search for words or phrases in the full text of the articles, produce a bibliography, and retrieve the text of promising articles. A link to the university's MELVYL MEDLINE system will allow users to search the entire MEDLINE database and then retrieve the full text of the articles using Red Sage. In collaboration with UCLA, part of the project will be to explore user behavior with electronic journals. This information will be used to develop a model for making such journals economically feasible. Various pricing schemes are being explored that include licensing fees for the university and user fees for printing [11]. Such partnerships are part of a growing trend, especially in academic institutions, where library and academic staff are coming together with commercial publishers, online utilities, and telecommunications and software companies to create an information environment that brings to the individual user a whole variety of resources both inside and outside the library walls.

Beyond Local Resources

Recent Advances

Once library users are equipped with all the necessary technology to establish remote access to their own library catalog or information system, suddenly a whole world of information opens up. During the 1980s, while many libraries, both private and public, constructed OPACs, some of the larger academic institutions began to provide access through their OPAC to the combined collections of all the libraries in their university system. Before long, other nonacademic libraries joined forces, so that union catalogs of many types of libraries, college, university, private, government, and special, became available by consulting one unified source. To add further value, libraries then began to add journal article databases, as well as a variety of other services and capabilities.

One prime example of the development and expansion of such a system is at the University of California (UC). In 1983, the UC Department of Library Automation implemented the MELVYL Online Catalog, now known as the MELVYL system, which provided bibliographic and location information on book and audiovisual collections in some seventy individual UC libraries located on nine separate campuses. Beginning with access through terminals located within most of the UC libraries, the system quickly became available to remote users via the UC network and by direct dial-up. Users could search for items in the entire database or limit their search to local campus resources. The size of the database increased tremendously, jumping from one million records in mid-1984 to six million at the beginning of 1992. This enormous growth was partially due to the addition of non-UC collections, such as the California State Library and the Center for Research Libraries. In the mid-1980s, other nonbook databases became available, beginning with CALLS, the California Academic Libraries List of Serials, which provided access to the periodicals holdings not only of the entire UC system but those of the nineteen-campus California State University system and the collections at the University of Southern California in Los Angeles and Stanford University [12].

A whole new service became available through the MELVYL system in 1987 with the addition of a five-year subset of the MEDLINE database. Similar features were used for searching MEDLINE as for searching the book catalog, with additional capabilities to take advantage of the sophisticated searching features of MEDLARS, such as exploding and starring terms. In this way, users familiar with the MELVYL catalog could easily make the transition to searching a journal article database [13]. MEDLINE was soon followed by Current Contents from the Institute for Scientific

Information (ISI), a series of databases from Information Access Company (IAC), and more recently several other databases made available through a reciprocal agreement with Stanford University. The system thus provided access to general periodical and newspaper literature, as well as to the specialized scientific and medical literature. With the addition of the USE command in the late eighties, the MELVYL system expanded its access potential even further. This capability provided a gateway to other library catalogs and databases, including the CARL databases in 1989 and a whole range of other systems in early 1991. Clearly the MELVYL system has developed into a tremendous resource for libraries and their users throughout the state of California. With the addition of the MEDLINE backfiles in early 1993, users are now able to search MEDLINE from 1966 to the present using MELVYL MEDLINE. The system has been an especially rich resource for health sciences library users with the holdings of some eight separate health sciences libraries at five separate UC campuses.

The 1980s saw extensive building of OPACs at institutions across the country, some limited to single collections, others providing holdings information for a variety of libraries of all types. At about the same time, some parallel developments were occurring which would allow for the linking of those resources and for access to them by individual users at local terminals. High-speed telecommunications links were being established not only on individual campuses but between remotely separated computer centers across the country, including wide area networks (WANs) such as the Internet. At the same time, protocols were being developed to allow different types of computers to communicate across these networks. The Internet, using the Transmission Control Protocol/Internet Protocol (TCP/IP) suite of protocols, now makes it possible for the thousands of mainframes and file servers that support OPACs to communicate with one another [14]. Anyone at a terminal with an Internet connection and applications programs such as the Telnet virtual terminal program can have access to remote databases mounted on any computer across the country [15]. Through the Internet, users located in a small town in the Midwest with few local information resources can have the same type of access as scholars at a large West Coast university. Begun in 1969 as ARPANET (Advanced Research Projects Agency Network) to assist communication between organizations involved in government-sponsored research, the Internet today links thousands of computers around the world and is used by individuals in private and public institutions, universities, community colleges, and special and public libraries. While the Internet has many capabilities, the remote log-in function that allows access to distant library catalogs and databases makes up a large percentage of network usage [16].

Today, over 200 libraries make their catalogs available over the Internet. These catalogs, however, are often the centers of much wider systems of information. The so-called campus-wide information systems (CWIS) usually include not only the local OPAC but many other locally mounted databases ranging from university catalogs, telephone directories, and commercial databases to the full text of reference works. The University of North Carolina at Chapel Hill, for example, provides access to the campus directory, job openings, and continuing education courses, as well as a series of bibliographies prepared by Health Sciences Library staff on AIDS topics and campus newsletters [17]. UNWIN, the University of Washington's Information Navigator, provides access to a variety of campus resources, including the Health Sciences Library's online catalog, a number of databases including MEDLINE and PsycINFO, a staff directory, online dictionaries, and an encyclopedia, as well as an events calendar and employment listings [18].

While systems such as these are invaluable to local and remote users, the size of the collections pales beside the rich resources made available through public utility systems such as OCLC. While long a staple for libraries to find quickly locations and transmit ILL requests, OCLC has traditionally been available only to library staff using dedicated terminals. With changes to their networking capabilities in 1991, OCLC provided more flexibility in accessing their services, including dial-up and Internet accessibility. In October 1991, a new OCLC service was introduced that made the identification and location functions of OCLC available to the end user [19]. FirstSearch was designed specifically for library users. Available through dedicated terminals in the library, or remotely through local networks or through the Internet, users can search the same enormous resources of OCLC's 14,000 libraries through WorldCat. One of the best features of FirstSearch is its ability to link a bibliographic record to the holdings of the local library, not only in the book collection, but in the various journal article databases that are being added to the system [20]. When users bring up a bibliographic record for a book or journal article, the system can immediately tell them if it is owned by the local library, as well as providing other locations in their state for the item they need. With over twenty-seven million records in the system and more than 460 million location codes [21], this is indeed a wealth of information for end users. Beginning in 1993, the MEDLINE database was added to those available through FirstSearch.

Individual and union online catalogs have proved a tremendous resource for librarians to consult for locations of items their library does not own. Now this same resource is available directly to library end users. Thanks to the networks, local and worldwide, users can have access beyond the walls of the library. Moreover, the location information is no longer just for books, but is increasingly available for journal articles as well, which is a particularly useful trend for health sciences libraries and their users. For example, the University of California has now added links between the CALLS database, which includes holdings information for the UC and other libraries in the MELVYL system, and the MELVYL MEDLINE database. As a result, when users complete their search and determine the need for particular references, locations of the specific journals are instantly made available with a simple command.

While location information has greatly added to the usefulness of these union catalogs, requesting and receiving documents from distant institutions can remain a problem for library users without assistance from library staff. Because of this, some of the larger, multi-institutional systems are being enhanced or designed initially to allow users to identify a necessary item, find a location, and then request the item, whether from the local library or from some distant institution, all from the users' individual terminals. The MELVYL system, for example, developed a document requesting function by linking the system with individual campus document delivery services. This function will enable registered users to retrieve a citation from the MEDLINE database or for a book at one of the campus libraries and immediately send an electronic mail request for the item to their own campus service. Requests automatically include location information so that the campus service can quickly direct the request.

The University of Maine System Libraries have also developed a "one key stroke" electronic requesting service through their OPAC. The union catalog includes holdings and location information for the seven campus libraries, the Maine State Library and Law and Legislative Reference Libraries, and the Bangor Public Libraries. Over eighty off-campus centers also have access to the database, though they do not contribute holdings. Registered users of any of these libraries are able to search the catalog, either for their own local resources or for the entire database of holdings. When users identify a book they want, they can immediately request that it be delivered to their local site. By invoking the "request" option, the system prompts them for their name, ID number, and any special instructions they might have. The system then verifies the user information and stores the request in the file of the library which owns the book. That library then retrieves the request, prints a paging slip, and pulls the item from the shelf. If a requested book is not available, the system also prints a notice for the user which is sent to the user's local library. Although the system only works for books, the university has plans to expand it to include journal articles and to mount IAC databases. The library which owns a requested item is responsible for packaging and sending it to the user's library. The borrowing library informs their user that the item is ready for pickup. The university libraries, however, provide a further service for their faculty by delivering the items to their offices by campus mail. Response to the system has been tremendous. Initially, there was some concern that public library users might overwhelm the system with requests for items from academic collections, but so far this has not happened. Since requests for items at other locations are integrated into user circulation records at the local library, regular circulation limits can prevent any potential overuse of the service. While all the larger libraries in the system are net lenders, some of the bigger university libraries have found that they also use the system heavily to borrow items that only the smaller libraries own. The delivery side of the service has proved to be expensive for the participating libraries, with staff time and mailing costs increasing significantly. In fact, the university has since switched from U.S. mail to a private delivery service between the libraries with the largest volumes of requested items, since this has proved to be more cost effective for delivery [22].

While the Maine system, at present, only works for books, OhioLINK has been designed from its inception with the ability to request items in any format held in any of the libraries included in the system. The network provides access to collections in thirteen state-assisted and two private university libraries, two medical college libraries, and the State Library of Ohio. Users are able to initiate requests for items at any of the sites. Most printed materials are delivered by a contracted delivery service, while articles and other smaller items are sent by telefacsimile. Since the system includes access to items stored in electronic formats, users also have the ability to receive electronically transmitted data [23]. Clearly, OhioLINK is filling the gap between easy identification and location and the rapid delivery of the information required. On a larger commercial scale, OCLC's FirstSearch has also developed a user-initiated requesting function. By establishing a link between FirstSearch and the ILL function, users are able to retrieve citations, get the holdings information, and send a message to their local library's file requesting a book or journal article.

Using the same basic concept, the UnCover system, the journal citation and document delivery service marketed by CARL Systems of Colorado and the Blackwell Group of England, allows users to request items directly using the Internet or direct dial-in access. (For further description of the UnCover system, refer to Chapter 3: Interlibrary Loan and Document Delivery.) Because of the efficiency of the system, by the time participating libraries receive their current issues of journals, article-level indexing is already available in the online catalog. With changes to the system in 1991, users can now order the complete documents for any articles included in the index. When an order is placed, the system searches the check-in records of the contributing libraries to determine which library has the journal and then transmits the request to that library. All the libraries that supply documents scan requested articles and transmit them to UnCover's headquarters, where they can be faxed to requesters. Scanned articles for which UnCover has publisher permission are retained in the system and reused for other requests; articles without retention rights are deleted. Users ordering articles can charge the costs, which include appropriate copyright compliance fees, to a major credit card or deposit account [24]. With some 20,000 titles included [25] and more libraries joining the system, the Un-Cover system is a major end-user resource for locating and requesting library materials.

By building in an electronic requesting function, systems like OhioLINK and UnCover have dramatically changed the role of both library staff and users. Users no longer need to come to the library to complete lengthy paper ILL request forms; library staff do not need to verify citations, search extensively for locations for requested items, or then send and keep track of multiple requests. All these functions are accomplished automatically by users and the system, sometimes from within the library, but more often from the office, laboratory, or home. In this new service paradigm, the library serves merely as a document supplier. Yet all these systems, though they may take users physically out of the library and place many of the traditional library procedures in their hands, still depend ultimately on the library collections to fulfill their function. ORION EXPRESS, OhioLINK, and UnCover are all library-based, so that the traditional services of selection, acquisition, cataloging, and maintaining collections are still vital to their success.

Collection-based systems for access and delivery of information such as those just described, while they represent a tremendous step forward, are limited in scope by the libraries which support them. To extend the resources to fill users' needs, systems such as OhioLINK, UnCover, and the MELVYL system were developed to provide access to multiple collections of different types of libraries. However, when users search these systems and request items, they are still requesting only the books and articles from journals that they know are owned by a particular library or group of libraries. For journal requests, in most cases, the articles themselves have been identified from other sources, print or online. To expand access for users, especially to the journal literature, some recent developments have provided links directly from bibliographic databases to networks of libraries or to commercial document delivery services. In this way, users can do their searching and requesting in one system, and they are not restricted to any particular library collection.

An example of this expanded access is the Loansome Doc function of Grateful Med which taps into an enormous network of health sciences libraries across the country and allows users to order articles directly from the results of their MEDLARS searches. (For further description of Loansome Doc, refer to Chapter 3.) Since Grateful Med currently enables users to search and request articles from the MEDLINE, HEALTH, or the AIDS databases, the most frequently used of the MEDLARS databases, this service provides truly comprehensive access to the biomedical literature. Moreover, being part of the DOCLINE system, Loansome Doc is supported by thousands of health sciences libraries throughout the country, including the collections of the NLM. With Loansome Doc, users no longer need to access their library's catalog to determine whether or not it owns particular journals. The automatic routing feature, linked to the data in SERHOLD, NLM's serials holdings database of over 3,100 health sciences libraries, means that the system, not the users, searches for the location of a title. Fees for this service are determined by the individual participating libraries and can include costs for copyright clearance when applicable. Suggested future enhancements should provide users with the ability to order documents from the retrieved citations from any of the MEDLARS databases available using Grateful Med [26]. Another possible revision would allow users to directly enter a citation for an item, have the system verify its accuracy through the online databases, and transmit the request to the DOCLINE library. Users now need to manipulate several menus and action screens to order the documents, which can be cumbersome; a future Loansome Doc capability could further utilize existing and developing technologies to ease the ordering process.

Loansome Doc is a good example of a system that provides that critical link between article-level bibliographic databases and direct document ordering from those databases by end users. Although it depends on filling requests from the collections of DOCLINE libraries, the system can hardly be described as limited since it can tap into libraries throughout the United States. The various systems set up by commercial vendors which also provide this type of link were, however, developed partly to compensate for library collection limitations, as well as the lack of article-level access in library catalogs. Linked as they are to the actual contents of a bibliographic database, commercial systems offer users the satisfaction of providing the entire contents of any reference retrieved through their searches. Such systems therefore rapidly deliver documents without users having to interact with a library.

An example of such a system is the Genuine Article from ISI. Established in 1966, the service began with a postcard mailed to ISI to order articles from *Current Contents* indexes. Now available online, articles identified from searching ISI's databases can be ordered electronically as well as by a variety of other methods such as telephone, fax, or telex. Another of the traditional database vendors, DIALOG (now owned by Knight-Ridder), also has a document ordering system called SourceOne which takes the concept of Loansome Doc one step further into the future. SourceOne enables searchers to order documents while actually doing the search by executing a command and naming a supplier. SourceOne provides the full-text document, including text and graphics for any document contained in the Ei Compendex Plus database. This function eliminates steps and switching from database to database or from function to function on a menu screen.

Other commercial vendors have developed systems that depend on this link between the bibliographic database and direct ordering of journal articles by end users. While some, like ISI, use their own supply of indexed journals, others depend on the products of secondary vendors. OCLC's FirstSearch and EPIC services, in addition to using the enormous resources of OCLC's WorldCat to provide document delivery, have also made connections with a large number of commercial document suppliers to improve search capabilities and expand ordering and delivery capabilities for the end user.

One such supplier, Engineering Information Inc. (Ei), provides subject access and document delivery for a specific scientific discipline and for more than just journal articles. Ei fills orders for full-text documents of virtually any article in the field of engineering from journals, conference proceedings, or technical reports. The journals and proceedings are indexed, abstracted, and included in the Ei Compendex Plus database. There is a basic fee for each requested item which includes copyright royalties.

Providing an extensive service, such as OCLC's FirstSearch, while it enormously expands the resources available to its users, poses difficult questions for a library. Does the library limit access to terminals in the library or provide remote access for its users? If remote access is available, how will staff train users, provide troubleshooting, and monitor use of the service? And, how much will all this cost? By offering a service with structured fees, libraries must be aware of the costs in light of budget constraints [27]. As the electronic document ordering capabilities advance into the twenty-first century, these and other questions pertaining to access, delivery, training, and economics will need to be asked, answered, and no doubt asked again and again as technology changes.

Future Trends

The various commercial and library-based services just described, which allow from a single workstation online searching and ordering from resources held at institutions spread all over the United States, are part of a growing trend toward the concept of "open systems." Such a concept is based on the idea of interchangeability, where a variety of hardware and software can be linked by a set of standard protocols so that the barriers between individual machines and between distant institutions are broken down. Data can thus be exchanged, using disparate machines and programs. Libraries have taken advantage of this concept and through the

Internet have provided access to increasing numbers of resources all over the world. The drawback has been the need for users to cope with a bewildering number of searching protocols. While access may be easy to all kinds of useful catalogs and indexes, learning their individual search language has proved an enormous challenge. The development of programs such as WAIS (Wide Area Information Server) has made search and retrieval easier, but their lack of sophistication remains a barrier.

Perhaps the best development for reducing this barrier is the concept of "client/server architecture," a fundamental element in open systems. With this type of design, the units in a system are entirely separate, acting either as the client, the requester of information, or as the server, the provider of information. Each unit can freely share information with any other unit since they all use a standard communication method [28]. For example, the client could be a bibliographic searching program mounted on a Macintosh workstation in a user's office; the server might be the cataloging subsystem mounted on a UNIX-based mainframe at the hospital library or a commercial database at the company headquarters across the country. The user could, by accessing such a system, formulate a search at the Macintosh, applying a familiar search program. The workstation (client) would then translate that search request into a standard format that is understood by the mainframe (server). The server would retrieve the needed information and package it so that it could be transmitted and sent back to the client where it would be translated into a format readily understood by the user.

The key to such a system lies in the standard format that allows the information to be sent from client to server and back again. Such a standard is Z39.50, also known as the linked systems protocol, approved by the National Information Standards Organization (NISO) in 1988 [29]. Developed initially to communicate bibliographic descriptions, it is now being adapted to support full text, including graphical images. Several commercial database companies and vendors of local library systems have begun to support Z39.50 in their products and to incorporate such compatibility in future services. This will have tremendous implications for libraries and their users in making all kinds of information easily available from the local workstation, all with a single search language and without concern for where that information comes from or how it is organized.

Various projects are already underway in linking systems with Z39.50, involving bibliographic utilities such as OCLC, library automation vendors, and university libraries. One collaborative effort is a project to link UC's IBM-based MELVYL system and the VAX-based system at the Pennsylvania State University. Another, Project Mercury, involving the Carnegie-Mellon University in conjunction with OCLC and Digital Equipment Corporation, is developing a complete electronic library, using Z39.50 as the central linking mechanism. NOTIS, a commercial vendor of automated library systems, developed a new product called PACLink, which connects one library OPAC to another using Z39.50 over the Internet which automatically processes document delivery and ILL requests. In a project with universities in Indiana and New York, users at each institution can search their own and any other linked OPAC, using their familiar local interface. They can directly request library materials, and all requests are automatically reviewed and approved before being sent on [30].

Electronic Delivery

Recent Advances

Technology has removed the necessity for users to visit or even telephone the library to determine whether needed materials are in the library's collection or in the collection of a library in another state or country. Moreover, technological developments have provided simple methods for searching these collections and for requesting those materials, wherever they might be located, without the assistance of library staff. Technology's final contribution to this new paradigm for information access and delivery is the ability to transmit the information directly to users again, eliminating visits to the library. Moving beyond the traditional methods of mail, courier, or, more recently, telefacsimile delivery, the information requested by users can now be transmitted in electronic form, with no paper copies.

A number of factors have helped bring about this phenomenon, most important of which are the developments in optical character recognition (OCR), image scanning, and mass storage devices. OCR technology has been available for many years, and recent improvements in software and scanners, along with the increase in storage capacity of personal computers and the proliferation of storage devices such as optical discs, have made it feasible and increasingly economical to convert large volumes of text into machine-readable text [31]. Coupled with the higher rates of data transmission over the Internet and better data compression, full-text storage and rapid transmission of entire books or journal volumes are easily accomplished. Such developments have begun to have a real impact on methods of information delivery.

While CD-ROM technology has been popular in libraries for some years, most of the early products have been either reference materials, like *Grolier's Encyclopedia*, or bibliographic databases, such as MEDLINE or PsycLIT. What made these CD-ROM products attractive to libraries clearly was their ability to provide searching capabilities with fixed costs, not their document storage capacities. Mixed-format discs were soon developed, such as MDX

Health Digest and Compact AIDS, which combine bibliographic references and the full text of several medical reference works or journal articles. More recently, however, CD-ROM products are being more heavily used by libraries as an alternative to full-text information, including entire journal issues. This new technology has been quickly embraced by all types of libraries, especially after the ability to network CD-ROMs and provide dial-up access to them alleviated the initial problem of single-user access.

While some products are merely disc versions of the print issue, others include complete indexing of the journals, providing access in one single disc. University Microfilm International (UMI)'s General Periodicals On-disc is a good example of a simple disc version of the print source; the paper product has been scanned onto an optical disc as an exact replica of the originals, including text and illustrations. This medium can certainly save shelf space and handling for libraries, but unless the disc is part of a network with multiple and remote access, the old problems of coming into the library and copying have merely been given a modern twist. Instead of photocopying an article, CD-ROM users now print it on paper with a laser printer. In the UMI product, since the indexing is not available on the same disc with the full text, users must consult another disc. Other products have combined indexing with the full text on a single disc, such as EBSCO's Magazine Article Summaries. Here, articles are stored as ASCII files, enabling users to search one disc which includes the entire text, indexing, and abstracts. Thus, users save time, and articles can be downloaded as well as printed.

Such a new product with yet a different twist, aimed specifically at health sciences libraries, is ADONIS. (For further description of ADONIS, refer to Chapter 3.) Made available in early 1992, ADONIS provides the complete text of approximately 600 journals in the health and life sciences, with data stored on a local library workstation [32]. The content of each article is stored as a graphic image and can be printed as it appears in the original journal, including all illustrative material. Searching is possible by author name, title words, journal name, or publication date, using Boolean logic. Most of the journals included are indexed in MEDLINE, and disc copies are received by the participating libraries within three weeks of publication. Because of the way the articles are scanned, the text cannot be transmitted electronically, so users again must either come to the library or use a local workstation connected to a local area network for access and delivery. While this may be a disadvantage, it can expand the number of journals to which the library subscribes. ADONIS is an on-demand, fee-based document delivery system that keeps track of all usage and calculates royalty charges. The system may be attractive to small health sciences libraries because the ADONIS annual subscription fee is far less that the combined subscription costs of all the journals included in the service. Moreover, it reduces the need and the costs for shelf space, binding, and handling. ADONIS allows libraries to increase their journal collections without contributing to the space problems that so many libraries face.

Although the digital storage of journal articles in the ADONIS system reduces the library's reliance on paper products, users must still cope with this medium, for ADONIS was designed for printing rather than online reading. Users need to print the articles each time they want to read them. If ADONIS is only available in the library, users need to come to the library to use the system. This limitation clearly conflicts with a growing demand for remote access to library services which more readily satisfies the information needs of users.

SAIL (System for Automated Interlibrary Loan), an experimental system project developed by the Communications Engineering Branch of the Lister Hill National Center for Biomedical Communications at NLM, offered such remote access and delivery. SAIL scanned and stored bitmapped images of journals and provided links between the scanned articles, the DOCLINE requesting system, and the MEDLINE citations. When a request was routed to NLM for a journal article for which a SAIL image existed, the SAIL workstation automatically received the request. Within minutes, the system either printed it locally for mailing or faxed the article directly to the user. While SAIL was only an experimental project, the implications for the use of such a system for document delivery are evident. The ultimate virtual library relies on access to full-text sources. In the health care field where speed of delivery can be a matter of life or death, developments such as SAIL to assist in document delivery are critical. These systems, however, raise issues such as copyright and licensing that need consideration before electronic document delivery systems can be practically implemented [33-34].

While SAIL used the DOCLINE-mediated interlibrary loan services as the source of document requests, it is recognized that many health sciences end users increasingly want direct access to document image databases. Moreover, they want rapid delivery over the Internet. These requirements have motivated the creation of DocView, a prototype system developed by the Research Engineering Group at NLM. DocView consists of Microsoft Windows 3.1-based client software and UNIX servers (both NLM-developed as well as public domain servers such as World Wide Web, Gopher, and FTP), which have access to document images. Using DocView, users can directly access these servers and retrieve over the Internet the stored images into their local workstations. DocView enables users to preview the document by displaying just the first page, zoom, scroll, cut and paste, electronically "bookmark" pages for special attention, print only the pages desired, and otherwise use the documents in a manner end users will want increasingly in the future. In addition to retrieving prestored images from databases, DocView lets users receive documents transmitted by Ariel workstations. Current developmental activities will be followed by a comprehensive evaluation of DocView [35].

Electronic information delivery completes the equation of remote, user-initiated access and delivery of information. Many of the systems described in this chapter have developed the capability of this type of delivery. Those such as OhioLINK and UnCover incorporate some type of electronic transmission of documents to their users. While this is a good beginning, at present the variety of full-text services can be complicated for libraries since all have their own unique organization, indexing mechanisms, protocols, and user interfaces. So far, there has been little cooperation among service providers to ensure uniform coverage. It will take a long time for an integrated solution to full-text online access to be found. Moreover, the demand for instant access to full-text information from these online systems and databases is not just for full text in ASCII format. Users require the entire text of a document, including graphs, charts, illustrations, and photographs, preferably in the same quality in which they were originally published.

As one response to the need for this type of transmission, the Research Libraries Group (RLG) developed a personal computer software package, Ariel, which in quality and speed is a real improvement over telefacsimile. (For a complete description of Ariel, refer to Chapter 3.) All types of articles, including photographs and half-tone illustrations, can be scanned and rapidly transmitted by the Internet to a user's workstation, where they can be printed on a laser printer or redirected to another workstation. Ariel extends the boundaries of library and commercial ordering systems into a new frontier of delivering electronically data and images to the workstations of users and eliminating the traditional methods of delivery including fax [36].

Yet another method for delivering the full text of an article, including all illustrations, has recently emerged in the form of the electronic journal. While the texts on CD-ROM products such as ADONIS are considered by some to be electronic journals, they do originate from the original paper journals. A new type of electronic journal is now being developed only in electronic form with no paper "original." A good example is the *Online Journal of Current Clinical Trials* (OJCCT) developed jointly by OCLC and the American Association for the Advancement of Science (AAAS) [37]. Designed to appear exactly like a print equivalent, OJCCT includes text, tables, and line drawings, though it cannot reproduce other types of illustrations. As a "true" electronic journal, the only paper copies of OJCCT are produced if users print an article at a terminal workstation or request a high-quality print from OCLC. Since this type of journal is designed with end users rather than the library in mind, libraries must decide how to provide access within their own institutions and whether or not they will offer ILL service. They will also have to consider how they will provide long-term access to this type of material if they are to fulfill their archival role. For end users, however, the electronic journal can be convenient, since with a personal subscription they can have immediate access and delivery at their own terminals. The one present drawback, the need for expensive hardware, will ultimately be eliminated as more sophisticated workstations become the norm.

Future Trends

Access to these electronic journals, both to the current issues and the archival files of back issues, may in fact be the key to whether or not they develop into standard resources in the future. While the number of these journals is increasing, they are still largely experimental in nature and may yet evolve into a very different format. Presently, access to them can still be a problem. Whether available by personal subscription, like OJCCT, or by online discussion groups such as Usenet, to be truly useful they must be searchable at the individual article level. Some of the traditional online indexing services such as ERIC have begun covering electronic journals, but the access they provide is merely to their titles, not to the full text of their contents. Some individual institutions have gone to the next step and have developed local system adaptations to allow searching of the full documents in these journals. A more comprehensive method would be to use the advantages of a client/server system to access electronic journals or any other machine-readable data, so that users with a variety of work-stations can be connected to remote files available anywhere on the Internet. Client/server- based information such as WAIS or World Wide Web, with their menus and other search capabilities and their easy document retrieval methods, are exciting new tools to help bring the expanding number of electronic resources to the individual's workstation [38]. With the advent of software such as Mosaic or Netscape, with their ability to retrieve a wide variety of media including sound and motion, the whole notion of information access and delivery is being completely rethought.

Publishers, anticipating how electronic journals and networking will affect them in the coming decade, are considering various innovative approaches to access and delivery of their products. TULIP (The University Licensing Program) is such an example. Designed by Elsevier, the program includes the loading of page images of materials sciences journals onto an Internet server for network distribution to participating universities. The universities are licensed to redistribute the articles throughout their campuses [39]. Apart from determining the technical feasibility of distributing journals over a network, the project also hopes to develop new and more effective models for journal subscription pricing and marketing so as to reduce the unit cost of information retrieval and delivery.

The Virtual Library: Implications for the Future

The various systems and services described in this chapter, which provide users with easy and rapid access and delivery to an enormous range of information resources, are the basis of a developing concept that is known as the electronic or "virtual" library, or the "library without walls" [40]. Though variously defined in the literature, the virtual library is simply a system that transparently connects individual users, in their home, office, or laboratory, to remote libraries and databases using the local library's network as a gateway [41]. Such a service relies on the existence of huge amounts of data, once available only in print, now stored on various devices at scattered sites linked by high-speed communications channels to be made available at the local workstation. These technological capabilities, coupled with ongoing reductions in library budgets and increases in materials prices and the developing sophistication of library users, have all played a role in this concept. The library now available to end users has dramatically expanded, with transparent access not only to the local library collection but to a vast number of other libraries' catalogs, to campus-wide information systems, and to library-based and commercial bibliographic databases. Linked to provide easy retrieval and document delivery, the virtual library has helped create quick and easy one-stop shopping for information for the end user [42].

This move toward a transparent information environment is already having an impact on libraries. As more information becomes available electronically, this impact can only increase as libraries move into the twenty-first century. The whole question of access rather than ownership of information will need to be addressed. If libraries find it more economical and efficient to provide access to information rather than acquiring that information, just what will their role be in the future? What will this mean for library materials budgeting and the traditional archival role of libraries? As client/server systems become more sophisticated, and users are able easily to access materials from local, national, and international sources, libraries will need to redefine their missions in terms of how best to serve their users and how most effectively to use their monetary resources. Will the monies available best be spent on books and journals or on the technology to access client/server systems? What effects will the cost of accessing and delivering documents have on the libraries' budgets? Or will the ease of access and the billing mechanisms of online document delivery systems, which allow users to charge documents to their credit cards, reduce the role of libraries in document delivery?

Whatever the future library's identity might be as it moves into the electronic age, clearly the traditional patterns of access and delivery will no longer meet users' needs. Current structures, standards, and procedures will all need to be constantly modified and recreated as technologies and the resulting capabilities change and as the costs of online access to information unravel.

Ten years ago there were few networks, little remote access to library catalogs or bibliographic databases, and no electronic journals or digital scanning of the journals. In another decade, access and delivery of information will look significantly different from how it looks today. Users will automatically initiate requests for items anywhere in the world from a computer either in the library or in their office or home or while in transit from New York to Budapest. They will access full-text databases and receive the items immediately or by fax. The documents received will contain not only text but high-quality graphics and illustrations and even sound and motion. Users will not need to learn different protocols because library systems all will be linked through client/server open systems using the Z39.50 system-linked protocol standard.

For libraries not to be confined by their walls, there are several issues that will need to be resolved so that quick, easy, and economical methods of information access and delivery can be provided. One of the primary issues is copyright, since the current copyright laws do not cover the many implications of electronic publishing. Although electronic access, especially through electronic journals, has improved the access to and delivery of information, as well as overall communication among scholars and researchers, the copyright laws have not kept up with the technologies and their implications for intellectual property laws. How are electronic journals best licensed, as well as print journals and commercial databases, as they become more readily available on the Internet? Who owns the information on the network, the user, the licensee, or the publisher or producer of the database? What happens to the concept of intellectual ownership when users can download ASCII material, make changes and upload it on the Internet, only for it to be revised by countless other users of the particular network?

Even if the most advanced systems for access and delivery of information are developed, they will be no better than the traditional methods if the laws and working arrangements that concern copyright and licensing are not addressed. The advantages of electronic access, speed, ease of use, copying, and multiple use, must not be compromised by outdated regulations. Copyright laws need to allow the copyright holders to be compensated without imposing cumbersome procedures for reimbursement.

When users need to wait for permission or have to pay unreasonable or high fees, they are more inclined to avoid or abuse the systems and to make illegal copies [43]. With all types of information being distributed electronically, the lines of ownership have changed. Possible conflicts of interest can arise if universities become involved in electronic publishing ventures by mounting electronic journals on their campus-wide systems. While companies such as DIALOG charge libraries and users each time that their databases are accessed, there are no charges each time users access the CD-ROM version of the same database. This imbalance also can affect charges for access to the more sophisticated electronic journals. Some publishers of electronic journals are very lax about copyright protection, being more interested in communication and distribution of the product. Mounting such a scholarly journal on a campus or hospital network may present certain obstacles since copying for noncommercial use by computer conferences, scholars, and libraries is permitted at no charge. Libraries, along with legislators and even society at large, will need to reconsider what intellectual property and fair use mean as commercial publishers move into the field of electronic publishing and assert their rights to copyright and intellectual property [44].

Library staff cannot alert users to the importance of compliance with the copyright laws in the same way they could with printed materials and photocopy machines. Users in today's library without walls will have access to electronic information at a multitude of workstations. They will be the ones to adhere to or infringe the copyright regulations. Establishing fair use provisions for electronic information is critical since libraries are in the lead in providing online information without charge to users. Librarians, therefore, need to communicate with the publishers about copyright of electronic information to provide reasonably priced and equitable access in these changing times. The library staff can monitor use of electronic publications only if they and the publishers agree on fair use of this information [45].

Another major issue related to the copyright implications of electronic access is licensing. Many license agreements which library systems or networks sign with publishers caution users of the electronic information that they can only download a portion of the database to a temporary file for research. These agreements pose questions especially when users build personal databases. What constitutes a portion of the database? How can shrinking library staff monitor the workstations located in the library? Adding in the remote access to networked databases, any control over what users download is virtually impossible.

Through cooperation of librarians working with publishers, licensing agreements for electronic information can be formulated. One concept recently suggested is electronic site licensing of journals. Although the foreseeable future will not witness the end of paper journals sold as sub-scriptions, arrangements must be made for the advent of electronic journals with virtually unlimited access in institutions and professional organiza-tions. The principle of a site license is a one-time, flat fee with no additional charges for normal distribution and use as defined in the licensing agree-ment. University systems, individual universities, regional or state library networks, and corporations that make the information available to those in their own organization seem to be appropriate candidates for such licens-ing agreements. What about the national companies that now repackage and resell information generally for profit, such as OCLC, CARL, RLG, EBSCO, and DIALOG? Is there a site license agreement for them? Some arrangement would need to be made for more than the flat fee, such as a per-use transaction since the specific information would be resold [46].

One advantage of electronic information networks for users is the idea that these networks can function as a publication mechanism, a way to express new ideas without preparing manuscripts for publication. The advantage, however, creates another major issue relating to ownership of intellectual property which tampers with the balance between the creators and users of scholarship and knowledge. This balance involves the fair use of copyrighted works for teaching, scholarship, and research [47]. As these new technologies provide ways for people to access, store, manipulate, and reuse information, a loss of control over the flow of information and its intellectual content could easily develop. High-speed telecommunications networks allow users to download hundreds of documents in seconds and create personal databases and totally new works and ideas from the data. A user in New York can access an electronic paper written by a colleague in Seattle, download the paper, add comments or arguments, cite several published scientific papers, and then upload the revision into the network. Another researcher in Florida can then access and download this docu-ment, make yet more revisions, and upload the new version. Who is the author of this work, considering that the two revisions may have substan-tially altered the original idea? In the past, copyright protected the intellec-tual ownership of the idea and the right to produce subsequent publications from the original idea.

Librarians in the decades to come will be involved in protecting the ownership of the information while encouraging optimum access to the information. How will librarians solve this information dilemma? Pres-ently, librarians need to raise the level of public awareness about the rights of intellectual property and to advocate legislation to strengthen govern-ment enforcement of intellectual property rights. Librarians also must be aware that commercial vendors will increase royalties for information access and delivery, thus the costs to libraries and their users, making decisions about budget allocations even more difficult. As the decade continues, librarians must be continually ready to make and revise decisions regarding collection development, as well as access and delivery functions, based on the resolutions to the intellectual property and copyright issues, the rapidly changing technology and its applications, and the escalating costs in information access and delivery [48].

Even today, some creators, contributors, and editors of electronic information advocate an approach to ownership that encourages the widest availability and the sharing of ideas. The electronic journal permits the authors to retain copyright and rights for reusing the information with the original source cited. Another philosophy is that the data is owned by the international community [49]. With these two very different theories, will anyone own any idea in the year 2050? Will there, in fact, be any copyright laws?

A final issue to be considered with the emerging methods of access and delivery is training for the library staff who will continue to need new skills and knowledge to manage a virtual library. Graduate schools of library and information science will need to develop new and innovative curricula to train the information specialists for the next century. Health information professionals will constantly need to update their skills and take advantage of educational opportunities not only in library and information science but also in computer and telecommunications technologies. Library staff at universities and hospitals will need to understand the intricacies of a network: hardware, software, advantages of campus-wide linkages, and the constantly developing technologies. With the flood of databases and document delivery sources, librarians will need to develop decision making skills to determine the best way for their users to access information and have it transmitted to them. They will need to decide what is more economically feasible for the library, subscribing to paper journals, subscribing to a CD-ROM service such as ADONIS, or obtaining licensure from a service such as TULIP to have the page images of journals mounted on a local network. Library staff will be involved in making decisions about the level of electronic access their institution is capable of sustaining in these times of changing technology and dwindling budgets. And with the growing resources available through the Internet, library staff will need to navigate skillfully this enormous source of information, to make it manageable for themselves and their users. These effects of technological change will no doubt continue into the twenty-first century as librarians continue to meet the challenges of change and maintain their traditional role in providing access to and delivery of information.

Conclusion

Information access and delivery, traditionally provided by libraries of all types, have undergone enormous changes in the past decade. Technological developments in computers and telecommunications potentially have placed most of the functions of access and delivery in the hands of the users. These developments also have removed the necessity for users to visit the library for their information, and they have laid the foundation for the virtual library. With such a development, the whole concept of what a library is or should be has been vastly altered. Libraries of the future will no longer be measured by the number of volumes added to their collections but by the amount of access they provide. Already a reality in one sense, the virtual library will not, however, soon replace traditional structures. Budgets and the technological capabilities of the institutional infrastructures cannot keep pace with the continual developments of the electronic age and its implications for information access and delivery. The vision of a virtual library with electronic access to unlimited resources is delayed by the administrative and economic support that would make such access a reality. New partnerships within an institution, among institutions, and between the library community and publishers still need to be formed in order to provide better ways of accessing and delivering information to the users who need it. Existing laws relating to copyright and intellectual property are slow to be examined and modified to meet the ever changing formats of publishing information. Resolving these and all the other issues that will arise with these new trends of access and delivery will make the journey into the twenty-first century an interesting and challenging one.

References

1. Malinconico SM. Information's brave new world. Libr J 1992 May;117(8):36-40.

2. Crawford W. The online catalog book: essays and examples. New York: G.K. Hall, 1992.

3. Matheson NW, Cooper JAD. Academic information in the academic health sciences center: roles for the library in information management. J Med Educ 1982 Oct;57(10,pt.2):1-93.

4. Ibid., 55.

5. Bellamy LM, Silver JT, Givens MK. Remote access to electronic library services through a campus network. Bull Med Libr Assoc 1991 Jan;79(1):53-62.

6. Ibid., 61.

7. Lindberg DAB, West RT, Corn M. IAIMS: an overview from the National Library of Medicine. Bull Med Libr Assoc 1992 Jul;80(3):244-6.

8. Roderer NK, Clayton PD. IAIMS at Columbia-Presbyterian Medical Center: accomplishments and challenges. Bull Med Libr Assoc 1992 Jul;80(3):253-62.

9. 1994 accreditation manual for hospitals. v.1. Standards. Oakbrook Terrace, IL: Joint Commission on Accreditation of Healthcare Organizations, 1993.

10. Schiller N, von Wahlde B. Toward a realization of the virtual library. ARL 1992 Jul;163:3-4.

11. DeLoughry TJ. Effort to provide scholarly journals by computer tries to retain the look and feel of printed publications. Chron Higher Ed 1993 Apr 7;39(31):19-21.

12. Moore JM. Also present at the creation. DLA Bull 1992 Spring;12(1):12-23.

13. Horres MM, Starr SS, Renford BL. MELVYL MEDLINE: a library services perspective. Bull Med Libr Assoc 1991 Jul;79(3):309-20.

14. Kalin SW, Tennant R. Beyond OPACs: the wealth of information sources on the Internet. Database 1991 Aug;14(4):28-33.

15. Nickerson G. Networked resources. Comput Libr 1991 Dec;11(11):38-42.

16. Farley L, ed. Library resources on the Internet: strategies for selection and use. Chicago: American Library Association, Reference and Adult Services Division, 1992. (RASD occasional papers no. 12).

17. Lloyd L. Campus-wide information systems. Acad Libr Comput 1991 Jun;8(6):7-10.

18. Ketchell D. Highlighting: University of Washington Health Sciences Library & Information Center. Supplement 1993 Mar;24(2):1-2.

19. Riehm SM. A first look at FirstSearch. Online 1992 May;16(3):42-53.

20. OCLC Online Computer Library Center. OCLC products and services for today's libraries. Dublin, OH: OCLC, 1992.

21. Mitchell J. OCLC interlending and document supply services; a review of current developments. Interlending Doc Supply 1993;21(1):7-12.

22. University of Maine implements statewide ILL. Libr Sys 1992 Jun;12(6):47.

23. Sessions J, Lee HW, Kimmel S. OhioLINK: technology and teamwork transforming Ohio libraries. Wilson Libr Bull 1992 Jun;66(10):43-5.

24. Lenzini RT, Shaw W. UnCover and UnCover2: an article citation database and service featuring document delivery. Interlending Doc Supply 1992 Jan;20(1):12-5.

25. Using Internet to UnCover... [advertisement]. MLA News 1994 Oct;(269):22.

26. Pacific Southwest Regional Medical Library Service. Enhancement 4: health professional access to DOCLINE: final report. Los Ángeles: University of California, 1988.

27. Kelly J. Computers in Libraries '92: what went on at this year's Computers in Libraries conference. Comput Libr 1992 May;12(5):18-9.

28. Phillips GL. Open systems and your library. Evanston, IL: NOTIS Systems, 1993.

29. Phillips GL. Z39.50 and the scholar's workstation concept. Inf Tech Libr 1992 Sep;11(3):261-70.

30. Nelson NM. Document delivery update. Comput Libr 1992 Sep;12(8):15-6.

31. Mallen E. Intelligent character recognition: it's not just recognition anymore. Bull Am Soc Inf Soc 1992 Jun/Jul;18(5):9-11.

32. Stern BT, Compier HCJ. ADONIS: document delivery in the CD-ROM age. Interlending Doc Supply 1990 Jul;18(3):79-87.

33. System for Automated Interlibrary Loan: system and operations description. Internal technical report. CEB/LHNCBC. Bethesda, MD.: National Library of Medicine, November 1992.

34. Thoma GR. Automated document delivery. Q Bull Int Assoc Agric Inf Spec 1992 May;37(1/2):84-8.

35. Walker FL, Thoma GR. Access to document images over the Internet. In: Proceedings of the ninth Integrated Online Library Systems Meeting, New York, May 1994. Medford, NJ: Learned Information, 1994:185-97.

36. Jackson ME. Document delivery over the Internet. Online 1993 Mar;17(2):14-21.

37. Keyhani A. The Online Journal of Current Clinical Trials: an innovation in electronic journal publishing. Database 1993 Feb;16(1):14-23.

38. Brandt DS. Accessing electronic journals. Acad Libr Comput 1992 Nov/Dec;9(10):17-20.

39. The TULIP Project: experiments in network delivery. DLA Bull 1992 Winter;12(3):24-5.

40. Mitchell M, Saunders LM. The virtual library: an agenda for the 1990s. Comput Libr 1991 Apr;11(4):8-11.

41. Saunders LM. The virtual library today. Libr Admin Manage 1992 Spring;6(2):66-70.

42. Troll DA. Information technologies at Carnegie-Mellon. Libr Admin Manage 1992 Spring;6(2):91-9.

43. Duggan MK. Copyright of electronic information: issues and questions. Online 1991 May;15(3):20-6.

44. Manoff M. MIT Electronic Journals Task Force report. Ser Rev 1992 Spring/Summer 18;(1/2):119-28.

45. Duggan, op. cit., 20.

46. Hunter K. The national site license model. Ser Rev 1992 Spring/Summer;18(1/2):71-2,91.

47. Young PR. National Corporation for Scholarly Publishing: presentation and description of the model. Ser Rev 1992 Spring/Summer;18(1/2):100-1.

48. Flanders BL. Barbarians at the gate. Am Libr 1991 Jul/Aug;22(7):668-9.

49. Okerson A. The missing model: a "circle of gifts." Ser Rev 1992 Spring/Summer;18(1/2):92-6.

Appendix A

Automated Circulation Functions

Blocks. Ability to deny library or registration privileges, both automatically by the system and manually by staff. System registration blocking needs to be interfaced with master files of the registrar or personnel office.

Cataloging on the fly. Ability to enter bibliographic records from circulation terminals.

Charge and discharge. Ability to charge or discharge (check out or in) items sequentially, with the system listing each item so that staff can see if they have missed any items; to charge materials to users of other libraries who are entitled to reciprocal borrowing privileges; to handle a variety of material types and items where one physical item does not correspond to one bibliographic entity; to handle variable loan periods (including hours, days, and weeks); to keep track of circulation status of specific items and categories of holdings.

Confidentiality. Ability to break the link between the patron and item identification once the item has been returned. *See also Security.*

Fees and fines. Ability to calculate automatically overdues fees and to view user's unpaid fines status; to keep history of library user fee status.

Hierarchical relationships. Ability to handle checking out a volume of a series cataloged individually and also listed on a serial bibliographic record. If the individual volume is shown as checked out, then the serial record must also have a charged out status. A similar situation relates to checking out a volume which has component part records in the database; both volume and component part records must have same charge status.

History or archival information. Ability to keep a history of charges, recalls, holds, and overdues on individual items and to see or get a report of this history. This information is useful for collection development purposes.

Holds. Ability to place holds on titles or specific copies of titles. Permit staff to determine which titles have holds, for whom they are being held, and after what date the material is no longer needed. Allow users to place holds from OPAC.

Interlibrary loans. Ability to accommodate interlibrary loans directly as a charge to a particular library; to record the charge and discharge of titles obtained on interlibrary loan from other libraries through a temporary record; to alert staff when checking in materials which do not belong to the library.

Inventory. Ability to wand each item on the shelf and have a report generated indicating which items are out of sequence, which items are checked out, and which items are missing.

Online public access catalog. Ability to determine quickly if a particular title or journal volume is checked out and the date due back without leaving the function one is using.

Patron file. Ability to enter user data from a circulation terminal; to have up to three addresses, with designation for primary billing address; to accommodate subject interest of users; to determine quickly for a particular user materials charged out, materials recalled or on hold, and outstanding fines; to keep and display to authorized staff a history of overdues notices, fines, and fines paid for the individual user; to link to the institution's master personnel and student databases.

Priority hold request. Ability to allow manual prioritizing or automatic prioritizing by user status as defined by library if there is more than one hold placed on an item.

Proxies. Ability to accommodate proxies. A proxy is a person who is authorized to borrow for another person, referred to as the sponsor. Ability to accommodate multiple proxies for single sponsor; to keep transactions by proxy but link them to sponsor; to tie proxy privileges to sponsor's privileges; to send overdues notices to sponsor.

Recall. Ability to recall an item that has been checked out; to generate recall notices and to apply fines if item not returned by new recall due date.

Renewals. Ability to see a list of items a user has checked out; to select items to renew; to have the option to renew all from a menu choice; to see the new due date on screen. If user is blocked, the system should flash message that renewal is not allowed.

Reports. Ability to generate daily overdues, fines, bills, recalls, and traces; to change wording of notices. *See also Statistics.*

Reserves. Ability to handle reserves as a location or permanent loan at the time of cataloging or subsequently; to accommodate short-term loan of class reserve items.

Searchable fields. From the circulation module, ability to search the patron file by user name or identification number and the catalog by call number, author, title, item bar code number, and, for reserves, also by course name and instructor.

Security. Ability to use password control for various levels of security by specified staff to access patron files and circulation records, to override blocks, or to change parameters.

Self-charge. Ability to allow users to check out materials on own.

Shelf reading. Capability to check sequence of call numbers or journal issues by bar codes.

Statistics. Ability to produce statistical reports automatically at specified time periods for number of charges, renewals, recalls, overdues notices, fines, items declared missing, and charges by patron status. Capacity to handle in-house use data collection by reading bar codes of material to be reshelved. Customized reports should be easy to program and to generate.

Traces (Searches). Ability to flag an item when it is not charged out and not found on shelf; to generate record of items the next day in shelflist order by collections.

Appendix B

Shelving Terminology

Case shelving. A type of shelving which is open only in the front. It may or may not have doors which can be solid, glazed, or wire grilled.

Conventional shelving. Standard steel library shelving, usually 90 inches high, double-faced, with seven adjustable shelves. *See Figure 2-8.*

Fixed shelving. Usually refers to conventional, standard steel shelving; nonmovable.

Linear foot (L.F.). The unit of measurement in which shelf capacity for the collection is expressed.

Nominal shelf depth or width. This is the dimension listed in the equipment catalogs, and it is the nominal size which is ordered. However, the actual size is usually 1 inch smaller than the nominally stated size.

Range. A row of connected shelving sections; can be either single or double-faced. An aisle separates one range from another.

Double-faced range. Two single-faced stack sections back-to-back. When facing the end of the range from the aisle, the left side is usually referred to as side A and the right side as B.

Section. The set of shelves between two uprights.

Stacks. A group of ranges. Also used to refer to the shelving area where the collection is stored.

Uprights. The vertical bars of metal shelving which support the shelves.

Appendix C

Shelving Measurements

ITEM	MEASUREMENT	COMMENTS
Aisle width - between ranges	>36 in.	
Aisle width - for wheelchairs	42 in.	required in some states
Base	3 - 4 in. high	
Book or journal heights	<11 in. (28 cm)	90% of research collections
Book width (avg)	1.05 - 1.11 in.	
Book volumes/linear foot (L.F.)	10.8	based on 1.11 in.
Journal width (avg)	1.42 - 1.73 in.	each library should determine own average
Journal volumes/L.F.	6.9	based on 1.73 in.
Capacity - functional	up to 66% of total L.F.	good for working purposes
Capacity - maximum	86% of total L.F.	stacks are considered full; impractical for working purposes
Floor load bearing weight - loaded compact shelving	300 lbs. per sq. ft.	

ITEM	MEASUREMENT	COMMENTS
Floor load bearing weight - loaded fixed stacks	150 lbs. per sq. ft.	
Oversize books or journals	up to 18 in. high >18 inches	can shelve upright shelve flat on newpaper shelves
Shelf depth for books	8 in. nominal or 7 in. actual	actual measurement is 1 in. less than nominal measurement used by manufacturer; other common nominal depths are 9, 10, and 12 in.
Shelf depth for journals	9 in. nominal	
Shelf depth for oversize volumes	>9 in. nominal 12 - 16 in. nominal	for upright shelving for flat shelving
Shelf depth for reference	10 in. nominal	
Shelf length (width)	3 ft. nominal	also available in other lengths
Shelves per section - books	7	in 90-in. high shelving
Shelves per section - journals	6	in 90-in. high shelving
Uprights, steel	90 in. high	also available in other heights

Glossary

AAAS	American Association for the Advancement of Science
AAHSLD	Association of Academic Health Sciences Library Directors
ACRL	Association of College and Research Libraries
ADA	Americans with Disabilities Act
ADONIS	Article Delivery Over Networked Information System
AIDS	Acquired immunodeficiency syndrome
ALA	American Library Association
ANSI	American National Standards Institute
APA	American Psychological Association
Ariel	Document transmission system (The Research Libraries Group, Inc.)
ARL	Association of Research Libraries
ARPANET	Advanced Research Projects Agency Network
Articall	Document delivery system (UMI)
ASCII	American Standard Code for Information Interchange
BACKFILES	BACK (older) citations of the MEDLINE file (database—NLM)
BIOSIS	BioSciences Information Services
BLDSC	British Library Document Supply Centre
BRS	Bibliographic Retrieval Services (InfoPro Technologies)
CAI	Computer-assisted instruction
CALLS	California Academic Libraries List of Serials
CARL	Colorado Alliance of Research Libraries
CATLINE	Cataloging Online (database—NLM)
CCC	Copyright Clearance Center
CCG	Conforms to Copyright Guidelines
CCL	Conforms to Copyright Law
CCML	Comprehensive Core Medical Library (database—BRS)
CD-ROM	Compact Disc, Read-Only Memory

CISTI	Canada Institute for Scientific and Technical Information
CitaDel	Citation and document delivery service (RLG)
CONTU	Commission on New Technological Uses of Copyrighted Works
CWIS	Campus-wide information systems
DIALOG	Online search service (Dialog Information Services, Inc.)
DOCLINE	Documents Online (NLM)
DOCUSER	DOCLINE User File (NLM)
DocView	Experimental document viewing system (NLM)
DPI	Dots per inch
E-mail	Electronic mail
Ei	Engineering Information Inc.
EPIC	Interactive online search system (OCLC)
ERIC	Educational Resources Information Centers
FastDoc	Document delivery system (OCLC)
FirstSearch	End user search service for access to the OCLC online catalog
FISCAL	Fee-Based Information Service Centers in Academic Libraries (ACRL)
FTP	File transfer protocol
F.Y.I.	Research and document delivery service (County of Los Angeles Public Library)
Genuine Article	Document delivery system (ISI)
GPEP	General Professional Education of the Physician
Grateful Med	User-friendly microcomputer based software for searching the MEDLARS system (NLM)
HEALTH	Health Planning and Administration (database—NLM)
IAC	Information Access Company
IAIMS	Integrated Advanced Information Management System (was Integrated Academic Information Management System)
ILL	Interlibrary loan
ILL-L	Interlibrary loan discussion list on the Internet
Internet	Network of networks using standard telecommunications protocol
ISI	Institute for Scientific Information

ISO	International Standards Organization
JCAHO	Joint Commission on Accreditation of Healthcare Organizations
L.F.	Linear foot
LIBID	LIBrary IDentifier (DOCLINE)
Loansome Doc	Document ordering feature of the Grateful Med software (NLM)
Locator	Client/server interface for Internet access to CATLINE, AVLINE, and SERLINE (NLM)
MAILMAN	Electronic mail system (Department of Veterans Affairs)
MARC	MAchine Readable Cataloging
MEDLARS	MEDical Literature Analysis and Retrieval System (database—NLM)
MEDLIB-L	Medical libraries discussion list on the Internet
MEDLINE	MEDLARS Online (database—NLM)
MELVYL	University of California online system
MHSLA	Michigan Health Sciences Libraries Association
MLA	Medical Library Association
MLAA	Medical Library Assistance Act
MUMPS	Massachusetts General Hospital Utility Multi-Programming System
NAILDD	North American Interlibrary Loan and Document Delivery (ARL)
NIH	National Institutes of Health
NII	National Information Infrastructure
NISO	National Information Standards Organization
NLC	National Library of Canada
NLM	National Library of Medicine
NN/LM	National Network of Libraries of Medicine
NOTIS	Northwestern Online Total Integrated System
NREN	National Research and Education Network
NSF	National Science Foundation
NUC	National Union Catalog
OCLC	Online Computer Library Center
OCR	Optical character recognition
Octanet	Automated interlibrary loan network (Midcontinental RML)
OhioLINK	Electronic library system for information services, resource sharing, and document delivery (Ohio)

OJCCT	Online Journal of Current Clinical Trials
OPAC	Online public access catalog
ORION EXPRESS	Document and book delivery service (UCLA)
OSI	Open System Interconnection
PACS-L	Public access computer systems discussion list on the Internet
PaperChase	End user online search system for MEDLINE (Beth Israel Hospital)
PRISM	OCLC communication software
PsycINFO	Psychological Information (database—APA)
PsycLIT	Psychological literature (CD-ROM database—APA)
QuickDOC	Program for offline data entry and ILL file maintenance in the DOCLINE system (Beth Israel Hospital)
RLG	Research Libraries Group
RLIN	Research Libraries Information Network
RML	Regional Medical Library
Romulus	Document ordering system (CISTI and NLC)
SAIL	System for Automated Interlibrary Loan (NLM)
SDI	Selective Dissemination of Information
SERHOLD	Serials Holdings Online (database - NLM)
SERLINE	Serials Online (database—NLM)
SourceOne	Document ordering system (DIALOG)
TCN	Title control number (NLM)
TCP/IP	Transmission control protocol/Internet protocol
TULIP	The University Licensing Program (Elsevier)
UC	University of California
UCLA	University of California, Los Angeles
UCSF	University of California, San Francisco
UI	Unique identifier
UMI	University Microfilm International
UnCover	Document ordering system (CARL Systems, Inc.)
UNWIN	UNiversity of Washington Information Navigator
Usenet	User network
VA	Department of Veterans Affairs (formerly Veterans Administration)

VALNET	Veterans Affairs NETwork
WAIS	Wide Area Information Service
WAN	Wide area network
WorldCat	World Catalog (databases — OCLC)
WWW	World Wide Web
Z39	Bibliographic standards for storing and retrieving information (ANSI)

Index

This is primarily a subject index. Personal authors of references cited in the text are not indexed. Acronyms and initialisms are given preference as indexing terms if more commonly used than full names of organizations or publications.

Author Biographies

Gretchen Naisawald Arnold has been a medical librarian since 1975 working in both hospital and the academic health sciences center settings. As a clinical librarian, she gained experience learning how clinicians use information. In her current position as Associate Director for Public Services at the University of Virginia Health Sciences Library, she is responsible for all public services operations including interlibrary loan and document delivery. The Health Sciences Library instituted a fee-based document delivery service at the UVa Health Sciences Center in 1988.

James Curtis is Assistant Director for Information and Education Services at the Health Sciences Library, University of North Carolina at Chapel Hill, and has been a health sciences librarian since 1980. He has extensive experience in public services administration, including the management of reference, access, education, and media services. Special projects with which he has been involved in his current position include the development of a fee-based document delivery service and the implementation and management of a networked electronic information service. He is currently heading a grant-funded project to extend computerized information resources and services to rural health care providers throughout the state of North Carolina.

Martha R. Fishel has been at the National Library of Medicine since 1976 where she currently holds the position of Deputy Chief, Public Services Division. Prior to that, she worked in the Library's Serial Records Section. She has been involved with the DOCLINE and SERHOLD systems since their inception in 1979/80. She worked with the Grateful Med development team in 1991 to formulate the document delivery portion of that program called Loansome Doc.

Beryl Glitz has served as Associate Director for the Pacific Southwest Region of the National Network of Libraries of Medicine since 1989. Before that she was a reference librarian at the UCLA Louise Darling Biomedical

Library, working in a variety of positions including Reference Desk Services Coordination, Interlibrary Borrowing, and Educational Services.

Susan Russell Lessick is Head of Research and Instructional Services at the Science Library at the University of California, Irvine, and has been a health sciences library manager in both hospital and academic health sciences settings since 1977. She has extensive experience in public services, including reference, access, education, and instructional technology services. She maintains an active interest in copyright developments as they affect libraries and has served on the Medical Library Association Governmental Relations Committee. She also chaired both the Medical Library Association Hospital Libraries Section, 1992/93, and the MLA/NLM Collaboration Task Force, 1993/95.

Carolyn E. Lipscomb is a consultant in Durham, NC. In nearly twenty years at the Health Sciences Library, University of North Carolina at Chapel Hill, she held a variety of positions, including Head of Circulation/Interlibrary Loan Services and Assistant Director for Human Resources and Communication. She also worked at the Library of Congress and has served as consultant to the National Library of Medicine, Institute of Medicine, and American University. She was a member of MLA's Task Force on Knowledge and Skills.

Irene Lovas has been the network coordinator at the Pacific Southwest Regional Medical Library since 1986 where she has been involved with the implementation of DOCLINE, NLM's automated interlibrary loan request and referral system, as well as the development and implementation of Loansome Doc, Grateful Med's document ordering capability. Before joining the Regional Medical Library, she worked as a medical librarian for the Veterans Administration in New York City and Long Beach, CA.

Valerie L. Su is Deputy Director and Head of Public Services at Stanford University's Lane Medical Library. She manages both information services and access services and serves as Acting Director as needed. She coordinated a major remodelling project, including the complete replacement of the library's stacks destroyed in the 1989 Loma Prieta earthquake, with minimal service reduction during construction.

N.J. Wolfe is Associate Director for Information Services at the Frederick L. Ehrman Medical Library, New York University Medical Center. He has been in medical libraries since 1981 with emphasis in public services and outreach. At Ohio State University he started the MHI (Medical and Health Information) Service which developed fee-for-service options for unaffiliated individuals at the Prior Health Sciences Library in 1985. In addition to fee-based services, Mr. Wolfe has expertise in facilities management and teaches a course *The Library as a Physical Plant* for the Medical Library Association.